The Evidence Based Medicine
Workbook

The Evidence Based Medicine Workbook

Critical appraisal for clinical problem solving

Robert A. Dixon BSc PhD
Senior Lecturer in Medical Statistics
Department of Public Health Medicine,
University of Sheffield, UK

James F. Munro BA MB BS MRCP MFPHM
Clinical Lecturer in Epidemiology, Medical Care Research
Unit, University of Sheffield, UK

Paul B. Silcocks MSc BM BCh FRCPath FFPHM
Senior Lecturer in Public Health Medicine,
University of Sheffield, UK

Butterworth-Heinemann
Linacre House, Jordan Hill, Oxford OX2 8DP
A division of Reed Educational and Professional Publishing Ltd

ℛ A member of the Reed Elsevier plc group

OXFORD   BOSTON   JOHANNESBURG
MELBOURNE   NEW DELHI   SINGAPORE

First published 1997

British Library Cataloguing in Publication Data

Dixon, Robert A.
  The Evidence based medicine workbook: critical appraisal for clinical problem
  solving
  1   Diagnosis   2   Clinical medicine   3   Diagnosis – Problems, exercises, etc.
  4   Clinical medicine – Problems, exercises, etc.
  I   Title   II   Munro, James F.   III   Silcocks, Paul B.
  616′.075

ISBN 0 7506 2590 2

Library of Congress Cataloguing in Publication Data

Dixon, Robert A.
  The evidence based medicine workbook: critical appraisal for clinical problem
  solving/Robert A. Dixon, James F. Munro, Paul B. Silcocks.
      p.   cm.
  Includes bibliographical references and index.
  ISBN 0 7506 2590 2
  1   Medical literature – Evaluation – Problems, exercises, etc.
  2   Medicine – Research – Evaluation – Problems, exercises, etc.
  3   Clinical medicine – Decision making – Problems, exercises, etc.
  I   Munro, James F.   II   Silcocks, Paul B.   III   Title.
  [DNLM: 1   Clinical Medicine – programmed instruction.   2   Problem Solving
  – programmed instruction.   3   Decision Support Techniques – programmed
  instruction.   WB 18.2 D621e]
  R118.6.D59
  616–dc20   96–24355
                                                                      CIP

Typeset by Keyword Typesetting Services
Printed and bound in Great Britain by The Bath Press, Bath

Contents

Foreword

Evidence based medicine, whose philosophical origins extend back to mid-nineteenth century Paris and earlier, is the conscientious, explicit and judicious use of current best evidence in making decisions about the care of individual patients (1). The practice of evidence based medicine (EBM) means integrating individual clinical expertise with the best available external clinical evidence from systematic research. By individual clinical expertise I mean the proficiency and judgement that individual clinicians acquire through clinical experience and clinical practice. Increased expertise is reflected in many ways, but especially in more effective and efficient diagnosis and in the more thoughtful identification and compassionate use of individual patients' predicaments, rights, and preferences in making clinical decisions about their care. By best available external clinical evidence I mean clinically relevant research, often from the basic sciences of medicine, but especially from patient-centred clinical research into the accuracy and precision of diagnostic tests (including the clinical examination), the power of prognostic markers, and the efficacy and safety of therapeutic, rehabilitative, and preventive regimens. External clinical evidence often supports current practice, but frequently invalidates previously accepted diagnostic tests and treatments and replaces them with new ones that are more powerful, more accurate, more efficacious, and safer.

Good doctors use both individual clinical expertise and the best available external evidence, and neither alone is enough. Without clinical expertise, practice risks becoming tyrannized by evidence, for even excellent external evidence may be inapplicable to or inappropriate for an individual patient. Without current best evidence, practice risks becoming rapidly out of date, to the detriment of patients.

The practice of EBM, then, is a process of life-long, self-directed learning in which caring for our own patients creates the need for clinically-important information about diagnosis, prognosis, therapy, and other clinical and health care issues, and in which we:

1   convert these information needs into answerable questions;

2   track down, with maximum efficiency, the best evidence with which to answer them (whether from the clinical examination, the diagnostic laboratory, the published literature, or other sources);

3   critically appraise that evidence for its validity (closeness to the truth) and usefulness (clinical applicability);

4   integrate the results of this appraisal with our clinical expertise and apply the result in our clinical practice;

5   and evaluate our performance.

Although this book focuses on the mastery of step 3, it integrates this step into the others by opening each exercise with a relevant clinical scenario and by prompting readers to specify three-part clinical questions and formulate appropriate searches for the best evidence. After guiding readers through the strategies and tactics of the critical appraisal of the evidence, it urges them to integrate that appraisal with their clinical expertise and make a clinical decision. Finally, by providing answers to the exercises, this book completes the EBM cycle by helping readers evaluate their performance.

This is a landmark text in the evolving field of evidence based health care, and will richly reward learners at every stage of their clinical careers.

David L Sackett,
FRSC, MD, FRCP (Ottawa, London, Edinburgh).
Professor of Clinical Epidemiology.
Director of the NHS R and D Centre for Evidence Based Medicine,
University of Oxford

1   Sackett DL, Rosenberg WMC, Muir Gray JA, Haynes RB, Richardson WS. Evidence based medicine: what it is and what it isn't. *BMJ* 1996; **312:** 71–2.

Introduction

The ability to read, understand and critically appraise research evidence is fast becoming a required core skill for clinical problem solving for many health professionals, including doctors, nurses and other clinical professionals, as well as health service managers and policy makers. Yet despite this, very few will have had any formal training or instruction in actually undertaking critical appraisal.

The key purpose of this book is to enable you to develop practical skills in clinical problem solving by reading and appraising published scientific literature, whether you are fully qualified or an undergraduate, and whether you are working alone or in a class. At the same time, the book will introduce you to some of the basic concepts in epidemiology, study design and statistics which you will need to do this. We hope that, in working through the exercises in this book, you will find that your confidence in reading research literature grows along with your ability to understand what the researchers have done, and why.

WHAT IS EVIDENCE BASED MEDICINE?

Evidence Based Medicine was pioneered in McMaster University, Canada, and, as a development of Critical Appraisal of Medical and Scientific Literature, involves the following steps:

- The posing of a problem in clinical medicine, usually in terms of a patient type, an exposure/intervention and an outcome.

- Searching of the literature through MEDLINE using a reproducible search strategy and limiting the number of articles through explicit criteria (e.g. restricting to randomized controlled clinical trials).

- Use of one of eight published study guides (therapy, diagnostic testing, overview, prognosis, causation/harm, clinical measurement, quality of care and economic evaluation) to assess the validity and extract the useful data.

- Assessment of the extent to which the preceding steps have provided a solution to the clinical scenario above.

HOW TO USE THIS BOOK

The body of the book is based around a series of nine research papers selected from the medical scientific literature. These papers have been selected not on the basis of being particularly good, or bad, examples of research, but simply because they suit our educational purposes in illustrating important points of method, and are short and clearly focused enough to make an exercise which can be worked through in a reasonable time.

The exercises are problem based. That is, each exercise begins with a clinical or policy problem and then leads you step by step through a paper which might help you solve that problem. The questions are designed to help you to read, extract information from, and critically examine the paper, with a view to deciding whether the research helps you to solve the problem you began with. Each exercise ends with a simple checklist to complete, which may help you to quantify your judgement about the paper. The purpose of the checklists is primarily educational, and we make no claim that they are a robust or well-validated method of assessing the quality of all published papers. Nonetheless, we hope you will find the checklists useful in making explicit the important features of other papers you read, and we have included a full set of checklists in an appendix for you to photocopy and use as you wish. If you are working within a group, differences in scores among group members will enable you to identify individual items on which there is not agreement. If working alone, you may wish to rescore some time later, with a fresh copy of the checklist to identify items on which you have given a different verdict the second time around.

In using the book, there are a number of points to bear in mind:

- Each exercise is self-contained, and you can work through the exercises in any order. Where appropriate, cross-references are included to relevant material in other exercises.

- We estimate that each exercise will take between 1 and 3 hours to complete, depending on how much of the material is new to you.

- Because the exercises use real (and unabridged) papers from real journals, you will undoubtedly come across some material which is difficult to understand at first reading (and perhaps at second and third too!); however, don't be put off – you will find that you can often decide whether or not a study's results are useful to you without understanding every detail of the method.

READING FIGURES AND TABLES

A recurring theme in the exercises is the need to interpret figures and tables before reading the results text. This is largely a matter of experience but guidelines (see Box A) and further reading can help. People differ from each other in their ability to construct and read tables, irrespective of their previous qualifications in mathematics and statistics.

Box A: Looking at figures and tables

I. Figures

Figures display and summarize the *broad* features of quantitative data pictorially. The most frequent types will be pie charts, histograms, dot-plots, box-plots, scatter diagrams and graphs (where points are joined by lines).

Look for:

- Self-explanatory title (who/what is depicted, from where and when?).
- Labelled axes.
- Clearly indicated scale type (arithmetic, logarithmic?).
- Scale breaks (where the scale on the axis does not start at zero).
- Units of measurement.
- Plot breaks or footnotes (e.g. when a new definition was introduced).
- Source of data.
- 'One message at a time':
  — Pie charts indicate the relation of parts to a whole.
  — Histograms, dot-plots and box-plots indicate the location, variability and symmetry of data. You can think of bar charts as 'histograms for qualitative data'.
  — Multiple box-plots, scatter plots and graphs also show how two variables relate to one another: Is there a trend? Is it increasing/decreasing? Is it non-linear (e.g. seasonal variation)? Scatter plots also indicate the variability in x and y; outliers (atypical values) may distort numerical conclusions such as correlation coefficients.

II. Tables

Ideally tables should be as simple as possible, with two or three small tables being preferable to a large complex one. Two-way tables (classified by row and column) essentially present the same material as graphs or scatter plots. Three-way tables are about the practical maximum.

Look for:

- Self-explanatory title with units of measurement.
- Clear labelling of rows and columns.
- Explanation of any codes or abbreviations.
- Row and column totals (if given, means or percentages may be more informative).
- Any natural ordering of rows/columns (e.g. by age? by income?).
- Numbers rounded to 2 or 3 effective digits.

III. Narrative summaries of figures and tables

When describing these, ensure that your summary:

- Is pitched at the right level (technical or lay audience?).
- Describes source and consistency of the data (see the footnotes and/or scale breaks).
- Aggregates categories if necessary.
- Describes overall trends, and notes subgroups where these do not apply.
- Avoids hyperbole and emotive terms.
- Distinguishes facts (e.g. numbers in table) from inferences (e.g. % change calculated from the table) from opinions/hypotheses (why the change occurred).

Note: Such narrative summaries are combined with summarized text to form structured abstracts, good examples of which are found in the *ACP Journal Club* and *Evidence Based Medicine*.

Where to find out more

Anderson AJB. *Interpreting Data. A first course in statistics.* Chapman and Hall, London, 1989
Chatfield C. *Problem Solving. A statisticians' guide.* 1st edn. Chapman and Hall, London, 1988
Fink A, Kosecoff J. *How to Conduct Surveys. A step-by-step guide.* Sage, Newbury Park, California, 1985
Tyrell M. *Using Numbers for Effective Health Service Management.* William Heinemann, London, 1975

**WHERE TO FIND
OUT MORE**

Evidence Based Medicine Working Group. Evidence Based Medicine: a new approach to the practice of medicine. *JAMA* 1992; **268:** 2420–2425.

Rosenberg W, Donald A. Evidence Based Medicine: an approach to clinical problem solving. *Br Med J* 1995; **310:** 1122–1126.

EXERCISE 1 A paper on clinical agreement

LEARNING OBJECTIVES

After working through this exercise, you should be able to:

A   Summarize and critically appraise a paper about clinical measurement.

B   Explain how the results in such a paper might apply to a clinical problem.

C   Perform and interpret simple calculations found in such a paper.

KEY POINTS

- Even 'experts' may disagree (especially if diagnosis is subjective).

- Kappa is used to measure agreement for categories (because agreement can occur by chance).

- Agreed criteria and measurement conditions can help to improve agreement.

CLINICAL RELEVANCE

To what extent can we expect second opinions to differ?

THE CLINICAL PROBLEM

You are a trainee in diagnostic histopathology. One morning you receive a specimen labelled 'Uterine curettings: products of conception?', obtained from a pregnant woman who has had vaginal bleeding with no evidence of a fetus on ultrasound. One possibility is that there has been a straightforward miscarriage with the fetus being lost before the scan; on the other hand, there is also the possibility of a hydatidiform mole (molar pregnancy), in which case she needs treatment and follow-up. When you examine the material under the microscope there is some hydropic change and trophoblastic hyperplasia, but you are not sure if this amounts to a molar pregnancy. You show the slides to one of the consultants in your laboratory, who says it is *not* a molar pregnancy, but who (confusingly) suggests you show it to the other consultant, who says it *is* one. Worried by this lack of agreement, you conduct a MEDLINE search and discover a paper, which you think may help you.

INTRODUCTION

Read the introduction to the paper, reproduced below, and answer the questions which follow.

In daily practice one recurring problem for histopathologists is whether products of conception show molar features or merely hydropic change associated with fetal death.[1,2] This is especially so for partial moles which may have fetal parts and membranes as well as villi, trophoblast, and decidua. There are, however, histological criteria that are said to easily distinguish between complete mole, non-molar pregnancy, and partial mole.[1-4] The diagnosis of partial mole or complete mole is important, with the patient having to enter the follow up surveillance programme for persistent trophoblastic disease and a request for her not to become pregnant; this entails measurement of urinary β human chorionic gonadotrophin for six to 12 months.[5,6]

This study was designed to test how good histopathologists are at differentiating complete mole, partial mole, and non-molar pregnancy, to assess the value of the recognized histological criteria.

1   In one sentence, identify the purpose of the study.

_____

_____

2   Why was the study felt to be needed?

_____

_____

METHODS

Fifty mixed cases of non-molar pregnancy, partial mole, and complete mole were selected from the files at Royal Preston Hospital and the Jessop Hospital for Women. Slides were coded and submitted to the seven participants. Some 12 months later, the slides were recorded and submitted for a second round. Table 1 shows the histological criteria sent with the slides. Ploidy studies were not carried out on these cases.

The results were then statistically evaluated for intra- and interobserver agreement as follows:

i   Consensus diagnosis—defined if greater than, or equal to, five pathologists agreeing for both runs;

ii   Interobserver agreement—κ value[7] calculated for each 'pair' of pathologists:

$$\kappa = \frac{P_o - P_e}{1 - P_e}$$

where P_o =   observed agreement
           P_e =   agreement expected by chance

values   1·0 =   perfect agreement
                     >0·75 =   excellent agreement beyond chance
                  0·4–0·75 =   fair to good agreement beyond chance
                     <0·4 =   poor agreement beyond chance
                        0 =   chance agreement only

iii   Intraobserver agreement—percentage agreement between two runs for each pathologist.

3   Where were the patients obtained from?

_____

4   Over what period had the patients presented?

_____

5   What proportion of specimens came from each hospital?

_____

6   Do you think that the sample of patients was typical?

_____

_____

_____

7   Why were the slides coded?

_____

_____

8   What do you think was the aim of the 12-month wait, followed by recoding?

_____

_____

Table 1 Histological criteria	
Non-molar	Grossly normal/few vesicles
	Often fetus/fetal parts
	Variable hydropic change
	Atrophic attenuated trophoblast
	Occasional syncytial sprouts
Partial mole	Normal volume of placenta
	Often fetus/fetal parts
	Small vesicles mixed with normal villi
	Variable hydropic change
	Variable trophoblast hyperplasia
	Circumferential proliferation
	Central cisternal degeneration
	Scalloping of villi with trophoblast 'inclusions'
	Some villi more normal with blood vessels
	Some small fibrosed avascular villi
Complete mole	Bulky uterus > dates
	Bunch of grapes grossly
	Rarely fetal tissue (if ever)
	Swollen avascular villi
	Variable trophoblast hyperplasia

9   Why were the histological criteria listed in Table 1 distributed with the slides?

_____

_____

_____

_____

_____

10   Who assessed the slides in the study?

_____

_____

11   How did the authors assess:

a   *Inter*-rater agreement (agreement between different doctors)?

_____

Box 1.1: Blinding

In any research it is always possible that the results obtained will be biased, that is, *systematically* wrong in a way that would occur again if the study were repeated using the same methods (as opposed to a result that differs from the truth on this occasion simply by chance).

Bias can arise at any point in a study:

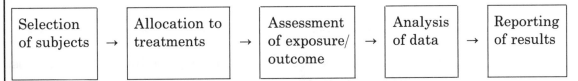

Bias in selection and allocation can be avoided by random sampling and random assignment to treatments, respectively. Assessment of exposure – for example by interviewers in a case-control study – may be biased if the person making the assessment knows whether the subject is a 'case' or a 'control'. Likewise, in a randomized controlled trial, the outcome may be assessed by doctors looking after a patient and their impression of the amount of improvement may, quite unintentionally, be coloured by their preconceptions of the efficacy of the treatments. The same considerations apply if the subjects themselves are aware of their diagnosis, or are asked about the effects of treatment.

This problem can be overcome by making allocation, treatment and assessments *blind*.

Blind allocation to treatment is when the person about to admit a patient to the trial is uninfluenced, in deciding whether or not to admit, by prior knowledge of which treatment the patient is about to receive.

Blind treatment is when patient and/or the health professional(s) involved in treatment are unaware of the trial treatment being administered, often achieved by use of elaborate placebos or 'double dummy' techniques. 'Single blind' implies the patient is in the dark, 'double blind' that both are! Ethical issues are not compromised as the patient must give informed consent to the process and the health professionals may be able to break the code in an emergency and record having done so.

Blind assessment is the assessment, without knowledge of treatment group, of outcome measures which may include base-line (on admission), mid-term (during treatment) and final (at end of or after treatment) measurements. If treatment is not blind, assessment may be kept blind by the use of independent assessors uninvolved with patient care, with precautions to ensure that conscious or subconscious clues are not communicated by patient or carers.

In observational studies blinding may be harder: if interviewers also, for logistical reasons, have to identify cases and controls they will not be blind as to the status of the patient; but one can try to interview patients before they are aware of their diagnosis.

We can extend the idea of blinding to include the statistician who, for example, should perhaps not know which group received active treatment and which the placebo, when analysing the results. If any biochemical tests are performed, there is a case that these too should be made anonymous. Lastly, while the individual writing up the results is not usually blinded, it is arguable that 'positive results please' and so again details of sponsorship, etc. should perhaps be kept hidden until the report is otherwise complete.

In short, the principle of blinding can be applied whenever knowledge or preconceived opinion may alter an assessment or measurement.

Where to find out more

Gore SM and Altman DG. *Statistics in Practice*. BMJ Publishing Group, London, 1982; pp 51–53

  b *Intra*-rater agreement (agreement by the same doctor on different occasions)?

_____

_____

_____

12 What strikes you as odd about your answers to the last question?

_____

_____

_____

_____

RESULTS

Table 2 shows the answers for each run. Only 35 out of the 50 slides achieved consensus. Table 3 gives the distribution of these cases. Of the 15 cases not reaching consensus, two were problems of differentiating partial mole from complete mole (cases 18 and 43). The other 13 involved the decision between non-molar pregnancy and partial mole. There was no problem in differentiating complete mole from non-molar pregnancy.

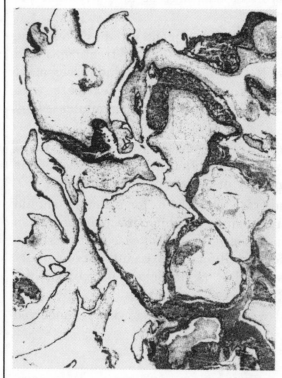

Figure 1 Complete mole showing circumferential trophoblast hyperplasia and swollen avascular villi.

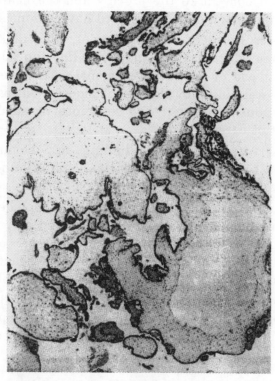

Figure 2 Partial mole showing villi with central cisternal degeneration, scalloping of villi with a 'Norwegian fjord' periphery, and mild trophoblastic hyperplasia.

Table 2 Histological opinions

| | Pathologist | | | | | | | | | | | | | |
| | A | | B | | C | | D | | E | | F | | G | |
Slide No	Run 1	2	1	2	1	2	1	2	1	2	1	2	1	2
1	NM	NM	NM	PM	PM	PM	PM	NM	PM	PM	PM	NM	NM	PM
2	NM	NM	NM	NM	NM	NM	NM	PM	NM	NM	PM	PM	NM	NM
3	NM	NM	PM	PM	PM	PM	PM	PM	NM	NM	CM	PM	NM	NM
4	NM	NM	PM	NM	NM	NM	NM	NM	NM	NM	NM	NM	NM	NM
5	NM	PM	NM	PM	NM	NM	NM	NM	NM	NM	NM	NM	NM	PM
6	NM	NM	NM	NM	NM	NM	NM	NM	NM	NM	NM	NM	NM	NM
7	CM	CM	PM	CM	CM	CM	CM	CM	CM	CM	CM	CM	PM	PM
8	NM	NM	NM	NM	NM	NM	NM	NM	NM	NM	NM	NM	NM	NM
9	PM	PM	PM	PM	NM	NM	PM	NM	PM	PM	PM	NM	PM	PM
10	PM	PM	PM	PM	PM	PM	PM	PM	PM	CM	CM	PM	PM	PM
11	CM	CM	CM	CM	CM	CM	CM	PM	CM	CM	CM	CM	PM	PM
12	NM	NM	PM	PM	NM	NM	NM	PM	NM	NM	NM	NM	PM	PM
13	NM	NM	NM	NM	NM	NM	NM	NM	NM	NM	NM	NM	NM	NM
14	NM	NM	NM	NM	NM	PM	NM	NM	NM	NM	PM	NM	NM	NM
15	PM	PM	PM	PM	NM	PM	PM	PM	PM	PM	PM	PM	PM	PM
16	NM	PM	PM	PM	NM	NM	NM	NM	NM	PM	NM	NM	PM	NM
17	CM	CM	PM	CM	CM	CM	CM	PM	CM	CM	CM	CM	CM	CM
18	PM	CM	CM	CM	PM	CM	PM	PM	PM	CM	CM	CM	PM	PM
19	CM	CM	CM	CM	CM	CM	CM	CM	CM	CM	CM	CM	CM	PM
20	NM	NM	NM	PM	NM	NM	NM	PM	PM	PM	NM	PM	PM	PM
21	PM	PM	NM	PM	NM	NM	NM	PM	NM	NM	PM	PM	PM	PM
22	NM	NM	NM	NM	NM	PM	NM	NM	NM	NM	NM	NM	NM	NM
23	CM	CM	CM	CM	CM	CM	CM	CM	CM	PM	PM	CM	CM	PM
24	NM	NM	NM	NM	NM	NM	NM	NM	NM	NM	PM	PM	NM	NM
25	NM	NM	NM	NM	NM	NM	NM	NM	NM	NM	NM	NM	NM	NM
26	NM	NM	NM	PM	NM	NM	NM	NM	PM	PM	NM	NM	PM	PM
27	CM	CM	CM	CM	CM	CM	CM	CM	CM	CM	CM	CM	CM	CM
28	NM	NM	NM	NM	PM	PM	PM	PM	NM	NM	PM	PM	PM	PM
29	PM	NM	PM	PM	NM	NM	PM	PM	PM	PM	PM	PM	NM	PM
30	CM	CM	CM	CM	CM	CM	CM	CM	CM	CM	CM	CM	PM	PM
31	CM	CM	CM	CM	CM	CM	CM	PM	PM	CM	CM	CM	CM	PM
32	NM	NM	NM	NM	NM	NM	NM	NM	NM	PM	NM	NM	NM	NM
33	NM	PM	NM	PM	NM	NM	PM	NM	NM	PM	NM	NM	PM	PM
34	CM	CM	PM	CM	CM	PM	CM	CM	CM	CM	CM	CM	PM	CM
35	NM	PM	PM	PM	NM	NM	NM	NM	NM	NM	NM	NM	NM	PM
36	NM	NM	NM	NM	NM	NM	NM	NM	NM	NM	NM	NM	NM	NM
37	NM	NM	NM	NM	NM	NM	NM	NM	NM	NM	NM	NM	NM	NM
38	PM	PM	PM	PM	PM	PM	PM	NM	NM	PM	NM	NM	PM	PM
39	CM	CM	CM	CM	CM	CM	CM	CM	PM	CM	CM	CM	CM	CM
40	NM	PM	PM	PM	NM	NM	PM	PM	NM	NM	PM	PM	PM	PM
41	CM	CM	PM	CM	CM	CM	CM	CM	PM	CM	CM	CM	CM	CM
42	CM	CM	CM	CM	CM	CM	CM	CM	CM	CM	CM	CM	CM	CM
43	PM	CM	PM	CM	CM	CM	PM	PM	PM	CM	CM	CM	PM	PM
44	NM	NM	NM	NM	NM	NM	NM	NM	NM	NM	NM	NM	NM	NM
45	NM	NM	NM	NM	NM	NM	NM	NM	NM	NM	NM	NM	NM	NM
46	CM	CM	CM	CM	CM	CM	CM	CM	CM	CM	CM	CM	CM	CM
47	NM	NM	NM	NM	NM	NM	NM	NM	NM	NM	NM	NM	NM	NM
48	CM	CM	CM	CM	CM	CM	CM	CM	CM	CM	CM	CM	CM	CM
49	NM	NM	NM	NM	NM	NM	NM	NM	NM	NM	NM	NM	NM	NM
50	NM	NM	PM	NM	NM	NM	PM	NM	NM	NM	NM	NM	NM	NM

NM: non-molar pregnancy; CM: complete mole; PM: partial mole.

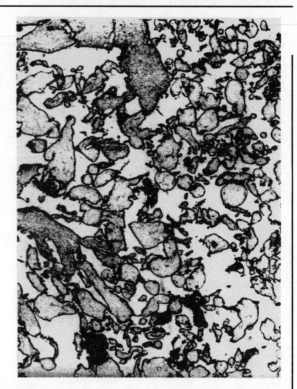

Figure 3 Non-molar pregnancy showing villi with mild hydropic change and no clinically relevant trophoblast hyperplasia.

Table 3 Distribution of diagnosis

Diagnosis	Number of slides with consensus
Non-molar pregnancy	17
Partial mole	4
Complete mole	14

Table 4 Kappa values

	B	C	D	E	F	G
A	0·589	0·690	0·745	0·670	0·586	0·595
B		0·491	0·658	0·455	0·417	0·561
C			0·773	0·563	0·578	0·501
D				0·618	0·628	0·599
E					0·466	0·459
F						0·393

Table 4 shows the κ values using data from run 1. Agreement varied between poor (pathologist F v G) to excellent (C v D). The values are for all 50 cases, including the 15 cases for which no consensus was established.

Table 5 Intraobserver agreement

	Agreement %
A	84
B	74
C	90
D	72
E	74
F	82
G	82

Table 5 shows the intraobserver agreement. The values are good to excellent, ranging from 72–90%.

13   **What do you think was the purpose of displaying Figures 1–3?**

_____

_____

_____

_____

14   **Using the data given in Table 2, can you confirm the authors' results in Table 3, using the definition of 'consensus' given in the methods section?**

_____

_____

_____

15   **What is the mean value of the inter-rater kappas given in Table 4?**

_____

16   **Complete the following table and calculate the value of kappa for observer A's intra-rater agreement.**

_____

_____

_____

Intra-rater agreement for Observer A (counts of observations from Table 2)

First reading (run 1)	Second reading (run 2)			Total
	Non-molar	Partial mole	Complete mole	
Non-molar	23	5	A = ?	28
Partial mole	B = ?	C = ?	D = ?	8
Complete mole	E = ?	F = ?	14	G = ?
Total	24	10	H = ?	I = ?

17   What are the 95% confidence limits for the kappa you have just calculated? Use the formula in Box 1.3.

DISCUSSION

About 15% of established pregnancies spontaneously abort; dilatation and curettage is often done in these cases to remove any retained products of conception.[1,2] When villi and trophoblast are present in the products of conception, the pathologist must exclude trophoblastic disease, especially complete mole and partial mole. Complete mole can be reliably distinguished from non-molar pregnancy. In two cases complete mole could not be easily differentiated from partial mole, but this is of little clinical importance as all molar pregnancies should enter the programme for detection of persistent trophoblastic disease.[5] Unfortunately (but not surprisingly), our study has identified problems differentiating non-molar pregnancy from partial mole. On review, it is clear that many cases of non-molar pregnancy showed significant hydropic change; the slides were purposely selected to show this feature. Nevertheless, some pathologists would be happy to leave these women and allow them to become pregnant again without follow up; others would impose restrictions on fertility, insisting on urinary β human chorionic gonadotrophin follow up. There are extensive histological criteria to avoid this problem (Table 1).[1-4] Each pathologist seems to feel as though he or she can use these parameters consistently, as shown by the good intraobserver variation (Table 5). These comments imply that either the histological criteria for partial mole are not being consistently applied among pathologists or that they are less than ideal for diagnosis. Our collective experience shows that in a non-molar hydropic pregnancy vesicles are hardly ever seen macroscopically. In partial mole one can see quite large (not small) vesicles mixed with normal villi. There is only mild trophoblast hyperplasia in most cases of partial mole and it is quite incorrect to say that there is hyperplasia of syncytiotrophoblast; syncytiotrophoblast is post-mitotic terminally differentiated tissue, incapable of mitotic activity. Recent studies with proliferating cell nuclear antigen support the low level of trophoblast hyperplasia in partial mole.[8] Other histological features, such as scalloping of villi and the presence of small fibrosed villi, are also seen in surgical terminations of pregnancy and are, in our opinion, unhelpful in differential diagnosis. The important feature in the diagnosis of partial mole is the *atypical* pattern of trophoblastic hyperplasia with a circumferential or multifocal pattern rather than the polar growth seen in normal first trimester placenta.

There are other diagnostic modalities that may help. Ploidy has been shown to be diploid in complete mole and frequently triploid in partial mole.[9-12] Non-mole pregnancy, if anembryonic pregnancies are included, shows a wide variety of cytogenetic and ploidy abnormalities including tetraploidy, trisomy, and triploidy.[13,14] Tetraploid and diploid partial mole however, have been described.[15,16] Assessment of ploidy involves either flow cytometry or static image analysis cytometry, both techniques being mostly unavailable in district general hospitals. Nevertheless, in cases where there is a serious problem in differentiating partial mole from non-molar pregnancy with hydropic change, sending some wet tissue or a block for ploidy studies might be prudent.

Box 1.2: Why bother with kappa for measuring agreement?

Kappa was devised as an index of agreement for *nominal* scales – that is, categories that lack a natural ordering: for example, different kinds of disease.

How is kappa calculated?

Suppose two GPs compare their diagnoses on 100 catarrhal children who attend their surgery. The doctors are raters, and their classification of patients as 'acute otitis media', 'acute tonsillitis' or 'non-specific cold' are ratings. The results might be displayed as in the following contingency table:

First doctor	Second doctor			Total
	Non-specific cold	Acute tonsillitis	Acute otitis media	
Non-specific cold	61	10	4	**75**
Acute tonsillitis	3	7	5	**15**
Acute otitis media	1	3	6	**10**
Total	**65**	**20**	**15**	**100**

The interpretation of this table is, firstly, that the first doctor considers 75% to have 'non-specific colds', 15% to have acute tonsillitis, and 10% to have acute otitis media, while the second doctor has rated 65% as 'non-specific cold', 20% as acute tonsillitis, and 15% acute otitis media. These numbers come from the row and column totals (also called marginal totals, in bold) for each category, divided by the total number of patients seen. Although the *overall* percentages are reasonably similar, they do not tell us how well the two doctors agree on *individual* patients.

For this we look at the cells on the diagonal running from the top left to the bottom right of the table (excluding the overall total, of course). These cells give the number of patients for whom the doctors agree about the diagnosis; in the table above, both doctors agreed that 61 patients had a 'non-specific cold', and the doctors agreed on the diagnosis in $(61 + 7 + 6)/100 = 74\%$ of their patients overall.

A problem with this observed proportion of agreement (denoted P_o) is that it makes no allowance for the amount of agreement there would have been if the two doctors had randomly classified their patients (in accordance with their particular marginal proportions). For example, the probability of a patient being diagnosed as having 'non-specific cold' by the first doctor is $75/100 = 0.75$, and the corresponding probability for the second doctor is 0.65. We would expect agreement on this diagnosis in $0.75 \times 0.65 = 0.4875$ of patients, simply by chance alone. If we apply this to the other diagnoses, and add the results, we can estimate the overall proportion of agreeing diagnoses that we would expect from chance (denoted by P_e).

In this example, $P_e = (0.75 \times 0.65) + (0.15 \times 0.2) + (0.10 \times 0.15) = 0.5325$. That is, we would expect agreement in 53% of cases.

Kappa is defined as the proportion of agreement in excess of chance, that is, the ratio of the **observed** agreement in excess of chance divided by the **maximum possible** agreement in excess of chance. If agreement is no more than expected by chance, kappa = 0. If agreement is perfect, kappa = 1.

This is expressed simply as: kappa = $(P_o - P_e)/(1 - P_e)$.

In this example, kappa = $(P_o - P_e)/(1 - P_e) = (0.74 - 0.5325)/(1 - 0.5325) = 0.44$.

Obviously, instead of comparing two different doctors (yielding an *inter*-rater kappa), we could compare a single doctor's assessments on two different occasions (yielding an *intra*-rater kappa, a measure of self-consistency).

Where to find out more

Armitage P and Berry G. *Statistical Methods in Medical Research*, 3rd edn. Blackwell Scientific Publications, Oxford, 1994; pp 443–447

Box 1.3: Interpreting kappa

Typically, values of kappa of 0·41–0·60 are regarded as moderate agreement, values of 0·61–0·80 indicate substantial agreement, and values above 0·80 are taken as almost perfect. An approximate formula for the standard error of kappa (which is needed to obtain confidence limits) when there are two raters is:

$$se(kappa) = \sqrt{\frac{P_o(1 - P_o)}{N(1 - P_e)^2}}$$

This formula is only approximate, although the inaccuracy falls as sample size increases. See Everitt (1968) for the mathematically preferable formula for two raters, which can easily be programmed into a spreadsheet.

Limitations of kappa

- Because kappa summarizes agreement, it misses patterns of agreement. It can therefore be useful to estimate kappas for each diagnostic category in turn.
- There are extensions to kappa that allow it to be applied to ordered categories, and also to the case where several raters assess patients (in which case the kappa is effectively an average of the kappas for each pair of raters). The same limitation applies, but the formulae for the standard error also become more complex, and bootstrapping (a computer-intensive method) has to be used.
- The value of kappa depends on the expected proportion of agreement, which in turn depends on the marginal proportions for each rater. These will themselves be related to the true prevalence of the diagnoses in the subjects being studied, so that a different case-mix will yield a different value of kappa, even with the same pair of raters; this means that variations in kappa values between studies can be hard to interpret.
- If you want to assess agreement of measurements (e.g. blood pressure), then a kappa-like index is available (the intra-class correlation coefficient). If there are only two raters, a simpler approach is to look at the *difference* between raters for each subject (Bland and Altman, 1986).

Where to find out more

Everitt BS. Moments of the statistics kappa and weighted kappa. *Br J Math Stat Psychol* 1968; **21:** 97–103

Fleiss JL. *Statistical Methods for Rates and Proportions,* 2nd edn. John Wiley, New York, 1981; pp 211–236

Dunn G. *Design and Analysis of Reliability Studies.* Edward Arnold, London, 1989

Diaconis P and Efron B. Computer intensive methods in statistics. *Sci Am* 1983; **248:** 96–108

Bland JM and Altman DG. Statistical methods for assessing agreement between two methods of clinical measurement. *Lancet* 1986; **i:** 307–310

What is the importance of an erroneous diagnosis of non-molar pregnancy being made when the 'correct' diagnosis should be partial mole? There are very few documented cases of persistent trophoblastic disease after partial mole; the incidence has been reported to vary from 0 of 51 cases of partial mole[15] to eight of 81 partial mole.[17] Even cases of choriocarcinoma consequent on partial mole have been described.[18–21] The risk is real, therefore, if very small.

There are problems with the routine diagnosis of partial mole. This conclusion is not novel.[22] It seems that histopathology alone cannot solve this diagnostic dilemma, but the situation may be helped by improving the diagnostic criteria for partial mole along the lines that we have suggested.

We thank Preston and Chorley Hospitals Research Fund for financial assistance.

Thanks also go to Ms M Jones, medical statistician, Northern Regional Health Authority, Newcastle upon Tyne, for expert statistical help.

18   What were the authors' main conclusions?

_____

_____

_____

_____

_____

19   What questions do you think are not answered by the study as presented?

_____

_____

_____

_____

20   Now write on a separate sheet of paper a structured abstract of the paper under the headings Aims, Methods, Results, Conclusions. Try to keep this to under 250 words.

The authors' abstract is printed below:

Abstract

Aims—To assess the degree of difficulty in diagnosing partial mole by analysing intraobserver and interobserver agreement among a group of pathologists for these diagnoses.

Methods—Fifty mixed cases of partial mole, complete mole, and non-molar pregnancy were submitted to seven histopathologists, two of whom are expert gynaecological pathologists; the other five were district general hospital consultants, one of whom works in Australia. These participants gave each slide a firm diagnosis of either partial mole, complete mole, or non-molar pregnancy. Some 12 months later, the slides were recoded and again submitted for a second diagnostic round to assess intraobserver as well as interobserver agreement. Standard histological criteria for each diagnostic category were circulated with the slides.

Results—κ statistics showed that complete mole could be reliably distinguished from non-molar pregnancy, but neither non-molar pregnancy nor complete mole could be easily differentiated from partial mole. In only 35 out of 50 cases was there agreement between five or more of the seven participants. Agreement between the expert gynaecological pathologists was no better than for others in the group. Interestingly, the intraobserver agreement for each pathologist was good to excellent.

Conclusions—These results imply that the reported histological criteria are either not being applied consistently or that they are lacking in practical use. An atypical growth pattern of trophoblast, rather than the polar accentuation seen in normal first trimester pregnancies, seems to be the important diagnostic histological feature for partial mole. Ploidy studies might also help with problem cases.

21   Compare the authors' abstract with your own version.

a   Do you think the authors' abstract is a reasonable summary
      of the results as presented?

_____

_____

_____

_____

b   Are there any claims in the abstract that cannot be confirmed
      from the paper?

_____

_____

_____

Does the paper help you with your problem?

22   So is the disagreement of your colleagues surprising, and how
      could it be reduced in future?

_____

_____

_____

_____

_____

_____

_____

_____

Title

Can histopathologists reliably diagnose molar pregnancy?   A J Howat, S Beck, H Fox, S C Harris, A S Hill, C M Nicholson, R A Williams

J Clin Pathol 1993; **46:** 599–602

Department of Histopathology, Royal Preston Hospital, Preston PR2 4HG   A J Howat and C M Nicholson

Department of Histopathology, Doncaster Royal Infirmary   S Beck

Department of Pathological Sciences, University of Manchester   H Fox

Department of Histopathology, Staffordshire General Infirmary   S C Harris

Department of Histopathology, Jessop Hospital for Women, Sheffield   A S Hill

Department of Pathology, Wangaratta District Base Hospital, Wangaratta, Victoria, Australia   R A Williams

Correspondence to: A J Howat

Accepted for publication 9 February 1993

References

1. Buckley CH and Fox H. Biopsy pathology of the endometrium. In: *Biopsy pathology series 14.* London: Chapman and Hall, 1989: 248–62

2. Elston CW. Gestational trophoblastic disease. In: Fox H, ed. *Haines and Taylor, Textbook of obstetrical and gynaecological pathology.* Edinburgh: Churchill Livingstone, 1987: 1045–78

3. Szulman AE, Phillipe E, Boue JG, and Boue A. Human triploidy: association with partial hydatidiform moles and non-molar conceptuses. *Hum Pathol* 1981; **12:** 1016–21

4. Szulman AE. Trophoblastic disease: clinical pathology of hydatidiform moles. *Obstet Gynecol Clin North Am* 1988; **15:** 443–56

5. Berkowitz RS and Goldstein DP. Diagnosis and management of the primary hydatidiform mole. *Obstet Gynecol Clin North Am* 1988; **15:** 491–503

6. Womack CC and Elston CW. Hydatidiform mole in Nottingham: a 12 yr retrospective epidemiological and morphological study. *Placenta* 1985; **6:** 93–106

7. Brennan P and Silman A. Statistical methods for assessing observer variability in clinical measures. *BMJ* 1992; **304:** 1491–4

8. Suresh UR, Hale RJ, Fox H, and Buckley CH. Proliferating cell nuclear antigen (PCNA) immunoreactivity as a means for distinguishing hydropic abortions from partial hydatidiform moles. *J Clin Pathol* 1993; **46:** 48–50

9. Benirschke K. Flow cytometry for all mole-like abortion specimens. *Hum Pathol* 1989; **20:** 403–4

10. Lage JM, Driscoll SG, Yavner DL, Olivier AP, Mark SD, and Weinberg DS. Hydatidiform moles. Application of flow cytometry in diagnosis. *Am J Clin Pathol* 1988; **89:** 596–600

11. Bagshawe KD and Lawler SD. Unmasking moles. *Br J Obstet Gynaecol* 1982; **89:** 255–7

12. Hemming JD, Quirke P, Womack C, Wells M, Elston CW and Bird CC. Diagnosis of molar pregnancy and persistent trophoblastic disease by flow cytometry. *J Clin Pathol* 1987; **40:** 615–20

13. Guerneri S, Bettio D, Simoni G, Brambati B, Lanzani A, and Fraccaro M. Prevalence and distribution of chromosome abnormalities in a sample of first trimester internal abortions. *Hum Reproduct* 1987; **2:** 735–9

14. Procter SE, Watt JL, and Gray ES. Cytogenetic analysis of 100 spontaneous abortions in North-West Scotland. *Clin Genet* 1986; **29:** 101–3

15. Lage JM, Weinberg DS, Yavner DL, and Bieber FR. The biology of tetraploid hydatidiform moles: histopathology, cytogenetics and flow cytometry. *Hum Pathol* 1989; **20:** 419–25

16. Lawler SD, Fisher RA, and Dent J. A prospective genetic study of complete and partial hydatidiform moles. *Am J Obstet Gynecol* 1991; **164:** 1270–7

17. Berkowitz RS, Goldstein DP, and Bernstein MR. Natural history of partial molar pregnancy. *Obstet Gynecol* 1986; **66:** 677–81

18. Gardner HAR and Lage JM. Choriocarcinoma following a partial hydatidiform mole: a case report. *Hum Pathol* 1992; **23:** 468–71

19. Looi LM and Siganesaratnam V. Malignant evolutions with fatal outcome in a patient with partial hydatidiform mole. *Aust NZ J Obstet Gynaecol* 1981; **21:** 51–2

20. Heifetz SA and Czaja J. In situ choriocarcinoma arising in partial hydatidiform mole: implications for the risk of persistent trophoblastic disease. *Paediatr Pathol* 1992; **12:** 601–11

21. Bagshawe KD, Lawler SD, Paradinas FJ, Dent J, Brown P, and Boxer GM. Gestational trophoblastic tumours following initial diagnosis of partial hydatidiform mole. *Lancet* 1990; **335:** 1074–6

22. Javey H, Borazjani G, Behmard S, and Langley FA. Discrepancies in the histological diagnosis of hydatidiform mole. *Br J Obstet Gynaecol* 1979; **86:** 480–3

Complete the checklist

Now use the answers you have already given to complete the following checklist and assign a score to this paper. There is space for you to add comments about the paper before you decide your final score.

If you wish, you can compare your score and comments with ours, which you will find in the answers section at the back of the book. If you have access to the World Wide Web (via the Internet) you can also compare your scores with those of other readers of this book. Details of how to do this are given in Appendix III.

The checklist is designed to be generalized to other papers of this type. A full set of blank checklists is included at the end of the book, which can be copied for use with other papers.

RATING SCALE 1 FOR ARTICLE ON CLINICAL AGREEMENT

		Ring the appropriate code			
		Yes	Unclear/ possibly	No	Not applicable
RESULTS					
1	Is the aim clearly posed?	2	1	0	N/A
2	Is it clear why the study was needed?	2	1	0	N/A
VALIDITY					
Subjects					
3	Is where they came from specified?	2	1	0	N/A
4	Is how they were chosen specified?	2	1	0	N/A
5	Is why they were chosen specified?	2	1	0	N/A
Raters					
6	Is where they came from specified?	2	1	0	N/A
7	Is how they were chosen specified?	2	1	0	N/A
8	Is why they were chosen specified?	2	1	0	N/A
9	Were they 'blinded' to other information?	2	1	0	N/A
10	If 'No', is method of presenting this information given?	2	1	0	N/A
Conditions of study					
11	Were Routine ('Normal' conditions) used?	2	1	0	N/A
12	Were the same conditions maintained throughout?	2	1	0	N/A
13	Was special training needed?	2	1	0	N/A
14	If 'Yes', did those who needed it, get it?	2	1	0	N/A
Statistical analysis					
15	Were methods used appropriate?	2	1	0	N/A
16	Were 'special' methods justified by authors?	2	1	0	N/A
Inter-observer agreement:					
17	Is reproducibility satisfactory?	2	1	0	N/A
18	Is the result adequately precise?	2	1	0	N/A
19	Was chance agreement allowed for?	2	1	0	N/A
Intra-observer agreement:					
20	Is reproducibility satisfactory?	2	1	0	N/A
21	Is the result adequately precise?	2	1	0	N/A
22	Was chance agreement allowed for?	2	1	0	N/A
Accuracy (i.e. vs 'gold standard')					
23	Was the 'gold standard' appropriate?	2	1	0	N/A
24	Is the result adequately precise?	2	1	0	N/A
25	Was chance agreement allowed for?	2	1	0	N/A
UTILITY					
26	Will the results alter my practice?	2	1	0	N/A

TOTAL (add ringed scores above): _____ **(A)**

No. of questions which actually applied to this article (maximum = 26): _____ **(B)**

Maximum possible score (2 × B): _____ **(C)**

OVERALL RATING (A/C expressed as a percentage): _____ %

COMMENTS:

EXERCISE 2 A paper on diagnosis/ screening

LEARNING OBJECTIVES

After working through this exercise, you should be able to:

A Summarize and critically appraise a paper on the diagnosis of disease.

B Explain how the results in such a paper might apply to a clinical problem.

C Perform and interpret simple calculations found in such a paper.

KEY POINTS

- Likelihood ratios help you combine sensitivity and specificity.

- Using multiple cut-offs allows you to make the most of available information.

- How do you know the prior probability?
  — Your hunch.
  — Characteristics of the patient.
  — Prevalence in the population.

- Generalizable to patient symptoms and signs, investigations and other diseases.

CLINICAL RELEVANCE

- How much will this diagnostic test tell me?

- Is this screening test any use?

THE CLINICAL PROBLEM

You are a GP working in a busy inner-city practice. The closure of many traditional industries in the area has meant rising unemployment in the local population and, you suspect, an increasing risk of alcohol abuse for many of your patients.

You know that there are many effective measures that can be taken to help people with a drinking problem, but you simply do not have the time to talk with all your patients at length, to find out whether they have such a problem.

How can you rapidly screen the patients you see, to identify those who might benefit from further help?

A POSSIBLE SOLUTION

An article you are reading about primary care and public health gives a reference to a study that may help you. You go to the library and look it up. But is the study valid? What do the results mean? And will it help you in practice?

This exercise is designed to help you answer these questions, and to learn how to apply similar methods to other papers on screening and diagnosis.

INTRODUCTION

Read the introduction to the paper, reproduced below, and answer the questions which follow.

The need for primary care physicians to detect drinking problems is becoming more compelling. Approximately 90% of adult medicine outpatients report using alcohol (1), and up to 45% report a history of excessive or poorly controlled drinking behaviors consistent with alcohol abuse or dependence (1–3). Alcohol abuse and dependence has important implications for the patient and the health care system. Excessive drinkers have an increased risk for injury, have multiple health problems (4–6), have double the mortality rate, and use health care services at higher rates than those who drink in moderation (7–10).

Physicians are in an ideal position to help patients with drinking problems. Unfortunately, this help is rarely realized because physicians detect drinking problems in as little as 35% of affected patients (2, 3, 11). Patients can be screened systematically for drinking problems with a simple yet accurate instrument (12). The CAGE questionnaire meets these criteria. The questionnaire was developed by Ewing (13) and was initially validated by Mayfield (14) in psychiatric inpatients. Bush subsequently validated the CAGE questionnaire using medical inpatients (15). The CAGE (acronym referring to the four questions, see below) asks only four questions: Have you ever felt you should *Cut down* on your drinking? Have people *Annoyed* you by criticizing your drinking? Have you ever felt bad or *Guilty* about your drinking? and Have you ever had a drink first thing in the morning to steady your nerves or to get rid of a hangover (*Eye-opener*)? Because the CAGE questionnaire has a sensitivity of approximately 80% and specificity of approximately 85% in medical outpatients (16–18), current recommendations suggest a 'cut off' of two affirmative responses as a positive screen for alcohol abuse or dependence.

There are two potential limitations, however, to use of the CAGE in primary care settings. First, no research has validated the CAGE against a structured clinical interview in a North American primary care population (19). Most of the studies validating the CAGE have used other screening questionnaires as the standard for comparison. Thus, the CAGE's accuracy, although assumed to be high, is unknown.

In addition, the current approach to interpreting the CAGE relies on the calculated sensitivities and specificities of various scores to determine the 'best' cut-off for a positive screen. In the context of screening, this score should capture the highest number of patients with disease (true-positives) while minimizing the risk for capturing patients without disease (false-positives). This goal is rarely accomplished by simply dichotomizing test results.

We investigated the alternative to dichotomizing the CAGE score, that is, assigning separate likelihood ratios for each possible score. We therefore propose to evaluate each patient according to his or her specific CAGE score.

1 Can you express the problem to be addressed in terms of:

a A patient type.

_____

b A measurement.

_____

c   An outcome.

_____

2   Briefly explain the purpose of the CAGE score.

_____

_____

3   What is your own CAGE score? If you are brave enough, compare your score with friends or colleagues.

_____

4   To be a useful screening test, what should the CAGE score achieve?

_____

_____

5   According to current recommendations, how should the score be interpreted?

_____

_____

6   In general terms, how might you go about finding out whether the CAGE score is a good screening test for alcohol dependence or abuse?

_____

_____

METHODS   The methods adopted in this study are given below.

We conducted the investigation between October 1988 and February 1990 at the Medical College of Virginia's ambulatory medicine clinic. We included as eligible for participation all English-speaking patients, age 18 or older, who were attending the clinic for a new or follow-up visit. Testers contacted patients as they left their intake interview with the clinic nursing staff and asked them whether they would agree to participate in a survey of the drinking habits of patients attending the clinic. Patients were assured of the confidentiality of the protocol and signed a consent form.

Immediately before the patient met with the physician, trained technicians administered the demographic section of the Composite International Diagnostic Interview—Substance Abuse Module (CIDI-SAM), the CAGE questionnaire, and the alcohol module of the Diagnostic Interview Schedule (DIS). The DIS was selected on the basis of its sensitivity, specificity, and predictive power for diagnosing alcohol abuse or dependence as defined by *Diagnostic and Statistical Manual of Mental Disorders-III* (DSM-III) criteria (20). Patients were tested only once during the study.

Data collected included the following patient demographic and clinical information: age, gender, alcohol diagnosis and symptoms on which the diagnosis was based, age of first onset of symptoms, and age of most recent symptoms. We defined a patient as having a drinking problem if the patient met DSM-III criteria for a history of alcohol dependence or abuse or the patient reported one or more symptoms on the DIS but did not meet criteria for a history of alcohol abuse or dependence.

To be consistent with the new DSM-III-R (revised) nomenclature and criteria for alcohol abuse and dependence, we converted DSM-III diagnoses to DSM-III-R diagnoses. We believed that this was important because some symptoms used in the DSM-III paradigm for alcohol abuse or dependence have been dropped from the DSM-III-R edition. We did this by including those DSM-III symptoms that also meet DSM-III-R criteria. Symptoms were talleyed for each respondent and a diagnosis was derived from the total number of symptoms. A total of one or two symptoms indicated a diagnosis of alcohol abuse whereas three or more symptoms were required for a diagnosis of alcohol dependence (21). The investigators then compared DIS-III-R diagnoses and CAGE scores.

We constructed a receiver operating characteristic (ROC) curve based on the CAGE'S performance compared with the DSM-III-R diagnoses. The ROC curve plots the true-positive ratio (sensitivity) against the false-positive ratio (1 — specificity) as the definition of a positive test is changed. The area under the ROC curve represents the test's ability to discriminate between disease and nondisease. A 'perfect' test gives an area of 1 whereas a worthless test gives an area of 0·5 (22, 23). In addition, we re-interpreted the data obtained by Bush (15) and by Mayfield (14), and constructed ROC curves for their data sets as well.

We calculated the likelihood ratios (LR) and confidence intervals (CI) for zero, one, two, three or four positive responses (24, 25). The equation for determining the likelihood ratio for a given test score is:

$$LR = \frac{\text{Probability of result given disease}}{\text{Probability of result for normals}} \tag{1}$$

The posterior odds that an individual with a given CAGE score has an abuse or dependence disorder is derived by multiplying the likelihood ratio for the CAGE score by the person's prior odds for having the disease. The equation for prior odds is:

$$\text{Prior Odds} = \frac{\text{Prior Probability}}{1 - \text{Prior Probability}} \tag{2}$$

where prior probability is synonymous with prevalence. Posterior odds can then be converted to posterior probability by the following equation:

$$\text{Posterior Probability} = \frac{\text{Posterior Odds}}{1 + \text{Posterior Odds}} \tag{3}$$

The posterior probability refers to the probability that the patient actually has the disorder in question given his or her score.

7   Who were the subjects of the study?

_____

_____

8   What measuring instruments were used to collect the data?

_____

_____

_____

9   What data were collected about each subject?

_____

_____

10   The CAGE score is being compared against a 'gold standard' for the diagnosis of alcohol abuse. What gold standard is being used?

_____

_____

_____

11   Suppose that, before you use the CAGE score, you estimate the probability that a given patient has an alcohol problem to be about 20%. This is termed the 'prior probability'. Using the information in equation (2) of the methods section, calculate the prior *odds*. (Refer to Box 2.1 to help you.)

_____

_____

12   Suppose that, after you have a patient's responses to the CAGE questions, you estimate the odds of an alcohol problem to be 0·6. This is termed the 'posterior odds'. Using the information in equation (3) of the methods section, calculate the posterior *probability*.

_____

_____

RESULTS   In Table 1, the authors present information on the study subjects

13   How many subjects provided data?

_____

_____

14   How many men were social drinkers? How many women were abstainers?

_____

_____

15   What proportion of men had any history of alcohol dependence or abuse? What proportion of women? What proportion of subjects overall?

_____

_____

Table 1 Lifetime Prevalence of Alcohol Consumption Disorders Using DSM-III-R Criteria among 821 Patients Attending a General Medicine Clinic*

Diagnosis	Diagnosis Determined by DSM-III-R Criteria		
	Men	Women	Total
	n(%)		
Dependence	113 (46)	89 (14)	202 (25)
Abuse	43 (17)	49 (9)	92 (11)
Social Drinker	76 (31)	346 (60)	422 (51)
Abstainer	14 (6)	91 (16)	105 (13)
Total	246 (100)	575 (100)	821 (100)

* DSM-III-R = *Diagnostic and Statistical Manual of Mental Disorders* (3d ed., revised).

16 What were the prior odds of a man in this population having any alcohol problem? How do you think this compares with your local population?

_____

_____

_____

_____

The authors present the CAGE score results for their patients in Table 2. Note that for a CAGE score of zero, the authors could have added 'automatic' values of 100 under 'sensitivity' and zero under 'specificity' to complete the table.

Table 2 Sensitivities, Specificities, and Likelihood Ratios Associated with CAGE Scores Attained by 821 Patients Attending a General Medicine Clinic

CAGE Score	Patients with CAGE Score		Sensitivity	Specificity	Likelihood Ratio
	Alcoholic*	Non-alcoholic†			
	n	n	%	%	
0	33	428			0·14
1	45	54	89	81	1·5
2	86	34	74	91	4·5
3	74	10	44	98	13
4	56	1	25	100	100

* Alcoholic = person with alcohol abuse or dependence.
† Non-alcoholic = person with no abuse of or dependence on alcohol.

Box 2.1: Probability and odds

Probability and odds are two ways of expressing our degree of certainty about future events.

The **probability** of an event is defined as the number of times we believe it is *likely* to occur, divided by the maximum number of times it could *possibly* occur. Conventionally, probability is expressed as a number between 0 and 1 (or as a percentage between 0 and 100%).

For example, if you throw an unbiased die very many times, it will, on average, show a four on one in six of all the throws. The probability of getting a four from a single throw is one in six, or approximately 0·167, or 16·7%.

The **odds** of an event is defined as the ratio of the number of times we believe the event is *likely* to occur, to the number of times we believe it is likely *not* to occur. Conventionally, odds are expressed as a ratio or fraction.

For example, out of six throws, our unbiased die is likely to show, on average, a four on one occasion and not on the other five occasions. The odds of getting a four are therefore 1:5, or one fifth, or 0·2.

Algebraically, if we denote the probability of an event as P, then:

probability that the event happens $= P$

probability that the event does not happen $= 1 - P$

so the odds of the event are the ratio of these two values $= P/(1 - P)$.

From this it is clear that, if the event is very unlikely (i.e. P is very small), then the probability and the odds are numerically very similar, because $(1 - P)$ is effectively 1.

Using the formula:

odds $= P/(1 - P)$,

it is easy to show that:

$P = \text{odds}/(1 + \text{odds})$.

Where to find out more

Bland M. *An Introduction to Medical Statistics*. Oxford Medical Publications, Oxford, 1987

17   Explain the meaning of the figures in the first three columns of Table 2.

Box 2.2: Likelihood ratios

The test characteristics of sensitivity, specificity and positive predictive value apply to tests which are dichotomous – in other words, which give results which are interpreted as being either positive or negative, with nothing in between.

However, many tests (such as the CAGE score, or a blood sugar test for diabetes) give a result which may be a single number from a range of possible values. If we simply define a single cut-off point and call everything below it 'negative' and everything above it 'positive', we are throwing away some information in the results which we might be able to use.

Instead, think of a test as providing us with new information which we can use to refine a judgement we have already made about how likely an individual is to have a given condition. Our assessment of this likelihood, which we make *before* the test, we call the **prior probability** of the condition. After we have the test result, we can make a better assessment of this likelihood, which we call the **posterior probability**. But how can we use the result of the test to take us from the prior probability to the posterior probability?

This is where **likelihood ratios** come in. When a test, such as the CAGE score, is validated, a likelihood ratio can be calculated for each possible result, or range of results, which the test gives. The likelihood ratio is defined as:

$$\text{Likelihood ratio} = \frac{\text{probability of an individual } \textit{with} \text{ the condition achieving the test result}}{\text{probability of an individual } \textit{without} \text{ the condition achieving the test result}}$$

The likelihood ratio relates the prior odds to the posterior odds using the following simple formula:

Posterior odds = Prior odds × Likelihood ratio

Note that this relationship applies to odds, rather than probabilities. This inconvenience means we have to take the additional step of converting our prior probability to an odds before using the formula, and the posterior odds back to a probability afterwards. The relationship between probability and odds is discussed in Box 2.1. To make this process easier for the busy clinician, a nomogram has been devised (Fagan, 1975).

Where to find out more

Fagan TJ. Nomogram for Bayes's theorem. *New Engl. J Med* 1975; **293**: 257
Sackett DL, Haynes RB, Guyatt GH, and Tugwell P. *Clinical Epidemiology: a basic science for clinical medicine,* 2nd edn. Little, Brown and Co, Boston, 1991; chap 4

18   What is the total number of alcoholic subjects? What is the total number of non-alcoholic subjects?

_____

19   What proportion of alcoholic subjects had a CAGE score of *exactly* 1? What proportion had a CAGE score of *at least* 1?

_____

_____

20   If you were to use a cut-off score of *two or more* as your
      threshold for suspecting alcoholism, as is currently recom-
      mended, what proportion of alcoholics would you correctly
      identify?

      _____

      _____

21   What term is given to this proportion?

      _____

      _____

22   Using the same threshold of suspicion, what proportion of
      people *without* an alcohol problem would you correctly
      identify?

      _____

      _____

      _____

23   What term is given to this proportion?

      _____

      _____

      Check your answers to questions 20 and 22 with the figures
      given in Table 2 to see if they agree. If you wish, you can check
      the sensitivity and specificity values given for other choices
      of cut-off in the same way.

24   What is the probability of alcoholic subjects answering
      exactly three CAGE questions positively? What is the prob-
      ability of non-alcoholic subjects doing this?

      _____

      _____

      _____

Box 2.3: ROC curves

The 'receiver-operating characteristic' (ROC) curve is a plot of how a test performs over a range of possible choices of cut-off point. It can be useful both in helping in the choice of a cut-off point, and in comparing the relative power of different screening tests. It gives a visual indication of the overall ability of the test to successfully discriminate between individuals with or without a condition, and of the implications of selecting a given value as the cut-off point for a test.

Each point on the curve shows the true-positive rate (sensitivity) and the false-positive rate (1 − specificity) for a single cut-off value. The latter will be (100 − % specificity) if the results are expressed as percentages.

If you were plotting an ROC curve for a test, you would take one possible cut-off point and calculate the proportion of individuals *with* disease who test positive (true-positive 'rate') and the proportion of people *without* the disease who test positive (false-positive 'rate') as a result. This would give you one point on your curve. You would do the same for other possible choices of cut-off point to give you the other points on your curve.

Note: There is a different definition of false-positive rate (see Box 3.3) which is inconsistent with the definition used here. You are therefore advised not to use such terms without first defining them.

A test which is no better than chance in discriminating between individuals with and without disease will have an ROC curve which resembles 'curve' B, below. A test which performs well in discriminating between such individuals will have an ROC curve which resembles curve A. The more sharply the curve deviates upwards and leftwards (i.e. the greater the area under the curve), the better is the performance of the test.

In choosing a cut-off value from an ROC curve, we will minimize the total number mis-classified by choosing the point on the ROC curve for which the vertical distance between that point and the 'line of unity' ('curve' B) is the greatest.

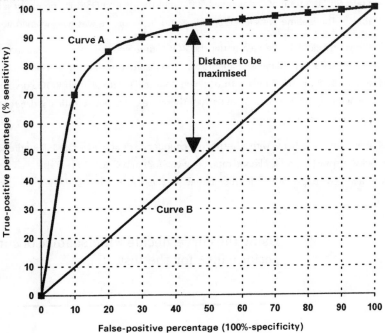

Where to find out more

Campbell MJ and Machin D. *Medical Statistics: a commonsense approach,* 2nd edn. John Wiley, Chichester, 1993; chap 3

Sackett DL, Haynes RB, Guyatt GH, and Tugwell P. *Clinical Epidemiology: a basic science for clinical medicine,* 2nd edn. Little, Brown and Co, Boston, 1991; chap 4

25   The ratio of these probabilities is called the *likelihood ratio* for this particular score. Calculate the ratio from your figures in question 24 and compare your result with the likelihood ratio given in Table 2.

_____

_____

_____

_____

26   Using the sensitivity and specificity figures in Table 2, plot the ROC curve for this test. A blank grid is provided overleaf. For more information on ROC curves, see Box 2.3.

The authors present an ROC curve for the CAGE test, and describe it in their results section. They also compare their ROC curve with those obtained by other researchers using the same test.

RESULTS

Eight hundred and thirty-six patients met inclusion criteria and were asked to participate. Of these patients, 821 agreed and were interviewed (participation rate, 98%). A total of 294 patients (36%) met the revised DSM-III criteria for a lifetime history of alcohol abuse or dependence (Table 1). The lifetime prevalence of abuse and dependence was 63% in men and 24% in women.

An ROC for our data is shown in Figure 1. The area under the ROC curve equals 0.89 with a standard error (SE) of 0·0128. This finding suggests a very powerful ability to distinguish patients with the disorder from those without it (22). The ROC curves for the data collected by Mayfield and by Bush are shown with our own. Mayfield's data give an ROC curve area of 0·91 with an SE of 0·0172 and Bush's data give an area of 0·90 with a SE of 0·0208. These areas are not statistically different and show a consistency of CAGE performance with various patient groups.

Table 2 shows the CAGE scores for the patients with a history of dependence or abuse by DSM-III-R criteria and for patients without such a history. The specificity, sensitivity, and likelihood ratio are given for each CAGE score. Table 3 shows the calculated posterior probability of an alcohol abuse or dependence disorder based on the CAGE score and the prior probability for an abuse or dependence disorder.

27   Using the curve, decide which choice of cut-off gives the 'best' performance for the test.

_____

_____

_____

_____

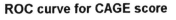

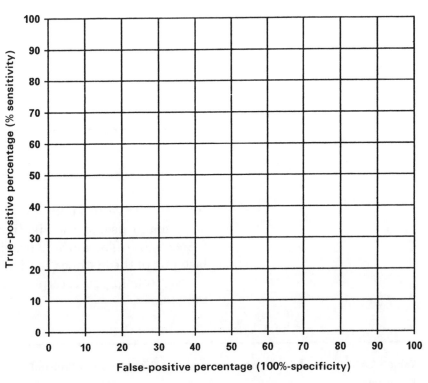

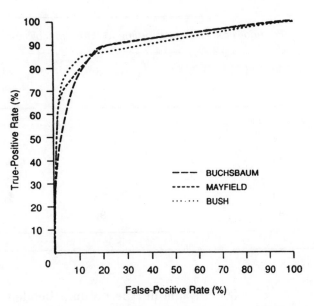

Figure 1 Receiver operating characteristic curves. Curves of CAGE scores reported in three groups of patients with the diagnoses of alcohol abuse or dependence.

28   In your own clinical practice, you may prefer to choose a different cut-off. What score would you choose and why?

_____

_____

_____

_____

29   Do you agree with the authors' judgement that the ROC curve
      suggests that the CAGE score is a powerful test for screening
      for alcohol abuse?

_____

_____

_____

An alternative to picking a *single* score as the cut-off point
is to make use of the likelihood ratio for each individual
CAGE score. The authors provide this in Table 3. Re-read the
last part of the methods section and then answer the questions
below, to help you interpret this table, which is not labelled
too clearly.

Table 3 CAGE Scores, Prior Probabilities, and Associated Posterior Probabilities for Alcoholism in a General Medicine Population

CAGE Score	Posterior Probabilities According to Prior Probabilities					
	10%	15%	20%	24%	36%	63%
	←			%		→
0	2	2	3	4	7	19
1	14	21	27	32	46	72
2	33	44	53	59	72	88
3	59	70	76	81	88	96
4	92	95	96	97	98	99

30   Examine the column headed '20%'. In this column, look at
      the figure on the row which begins with a CAGE score of 3.
      Explain the meaning of the figure '76' which you find there.

_____

_____

_____

_____

31   Examine the column headed '36%'. Using the likelihood ratios given in Table 2, verify each of the posterior probabilities in this column.

_____

_____

_____

_____

_____

32   Suppose the prevalence of alcohol problems among women in your community is 28%. A patient gives a CAGE score of 1. What is the probability she has an alcohol problem?

_____

_____

_____

_____

33   At what posterior probability might you consider:

a   Counselling?

_____

_____

_____

b   Advising the patient not to drive?

_____

_____

_____

DISCUSSION   Now read the investigators' discussion of their results.

We found that the CAGE performed remarkably well in correctly identifying medical outpatients diagnosed with alcohol abuse or dependence by DSM-III-R criteria. Our findings are consistent with those of both Mayfield and Bush for patients hospitalized on psychiatric and medical services (14, 15). This similarity in performance is particularly impressive given that the three investigations used different diagnostic standards to establish a diagnosis.

In conjunction with its power to discriminate between positive and negative patients, the CAGE offers the clinician the ability to define a given patient's risk for alcohol abuse and alcoholism based on his or her score. This is particularly important in groups where the prior probability of drinking problems is high. For example, in our group we found that using the conventional cut-off of two positive responses as a positive CAGE resulted in the automatic rejection of 78 (26%) of our DIS-positive patients with scores of 0 or 1. Yet, as shown in Table 3, a score of 1 was associated with a 46% posterior probability of abuse or dependence for all patients in our group and a 76% probability for men. This re-interpretation of the CAGE will influence our decision to pursue the diagnosis of dependence or alcohol abuse in our group (26).

Moreover, using likelihood ratios to interpret the CAGE scores enables the clinician to stratify patients along a continuum of risk for abuse or dependence: the higher the score, the greater the probability of a disorder. Thus, the patient with a score of 3 is at greater risk than a patient with a score of 2, and a patient with a score of 4 is at greater risk than a patient with a score of 3. Again, in a dichotomous model, all patients above a chosen cut-off are assigned the same risk. To simplify the process of estimating posterior probabilities for alcohol abuse or dependence in a patient with a given CAGE score, a nomogram such as that developed by Fagan can be used (27).

Several issues must be addressed with regard to our findings. First, although we chose the DIS as our 'gold standard,' we recognize that it is not perfect when compared with in-depth psychiatric interviews (28). We are encouraged that the CAGE consistently identifies patients at risk for a serious drinking disorder regardless of the setting and criteria used to make a diagnosis. This point strongly argues in favor of the discriminating ability of the CAGE.

Second, to interpret the CAGE by using likelihood ratios the clinician must have a reasonable estimate of the patient's prior probability for excessive or uncontrolled drinking. In this regard, prevalence data are available for different primary care settings, and the clinician can estimate risk based on data derived from settings that are similar to his or her own.

As this study shows and others re-inforce (29, 30), translating test scores into quantitative likelihood ratios enhances the richness of the information available to the physician. We believe that this approach facilitates the difficult task of making clinical decisions based on what appears to be limited information. We also believe this approach will help the physician identify more effectively patients who are having problems with alcohol consumption.

Grant Support: By the Commonwealth Center on Drug Abuse Faculty Grant Program and The Bureau of Health Professions HRSA Grant for Residency Training in General Internal Medicine.

Requests for Reprints: David Buchsbaum, MD, MHA, Medical College of Virginia, Box 102, Richmond, VA 23298.

Current Author Addresses: Drs. Buchsbaum and Centor and Ms. Buchanan: Medical College of Virginia, Box 102, Richmond, VA 23298.
Dr. Schnoll: Medical College of Virginia, Box 109, Richmond, VA 23298.
Dr. Lawton: Virginia Commonwealth University, Box 2030, Richmond, VA 23220.

34   How do the authors suggest you estimate the prior probability of alcoholism? Do you think their suggestion is reasonable?

_____

_____

35   You have seen that it is possible either to interpret test results using a single cut-point, or to use the likelihood ratios for each individual score. Which approach do the authors of this paper favour? What reasons do they give?

      _____

      _____

      _____

Does the paper help you with your problem?

36   What is the *main* conclusion of the study?

      _____

37   Overall, do you think the main conclusion is supported by the evidence?

      _____

38   What factors would you want to consider in deciding whether you can apply the main conclusion to your own situation?

      _____

      _____

39   Has the paper helped to solve the problem you started with?

      _____

      _____

The authors' summary of this paper is given below:

SUMMARY

■ *Objective:* To assess the performance of the CAGE (acronym referring to four questions, see below) questionnaire in discriminating between medicine outpatients with and without an alcohol abuse or dependence disorder.

■ *Design:* A cross-sectional design of a sample of consecutive patients who received both the alcohol module of the diagnostic interview schedule and the CAGE (Cut down, Annoyed, Guilty, Eye-opener) screening questionnaire.

■ *Setting:* The outpatient medical practice of an urban university teaching hospital.

■ *Patients:* All patients 18 years or older who signed a consent form approved by the university's institutional review board.

■ *Measurement:* Calculation of the sensitivity, specificity, receiver operating characteristic (ROC) curve, and likelihood ratio for CAGE scores of 0 to 4.

■ *Results:* Thirty-six percent of the sample group met criteria for a history of alcohol abuse or dependence. A CAGE score of 2 or more was associated with a sensitivity and specificity of 74% and 91%. The calculated area under the ROC curve was 0·89, whereas the likelihood ratios for CAGE scores of 0 to 4 were 0·14, 1·5, 4·5, 13, and 100, respectively. These ratios were associated with posterior probabilities for an abuse or dependence disorder of 7%, 46%, 72%, 88%, and 98%, respectively.

■ *Conclusion:* Clinicians can improve their ability to estimate a patient's risk for an alcohol abuse or dependence disorder using likelihood ratios for CAGE scores.

Title

Screening for Alcohol Abuse Using CAGE Scores and Likelihood Ratios   David G. Buchsbaum, MD, MHA; Robin G. Buchanan, BA; Robert M. Centor, MD; Sidney H. Schnoll, MD, PhD; and Marcia J. Lawton, PhD

Annals of Internal Medicine. 1991; **115:**774–777.

From the Medical College of Virginia and Virginia Commonwealth University. For current author addresses, see end of text.

© 1991 American College of Physicians

References

1. Buchsbaum DG, Buchanan RG, Lawton MJ, and Schnoll SH Alcohol consumption patterns in a primary care population. *Alcohol Alcohol* 1991; **2:** 215–20

2. Cleary PD, Miller M, Bush BT, Warburg MM, Delbanco TL, and Aronson MD. Prevalence and recognition of alcohol abuse in a primary care population. *Am J Med* 1988; **85:** 466–71

3. Coulehan JL, Zettler-Segal M, Block M, McClelland M, and Schulberg HC. Recognition of alcoholism and substance abuse in primary care patients. *Arch Intern Med* 1987; **147:** 349–52

4. Puddy IB, Beilin LJ, and Vandongen R. Regular alcohol use raises blood pressure in treated hypertension subjects. A randomized controlled trial. *Lancet* 1987; **1:** 647–51

5. Skinner HA, Holt S, Schuller R, Roy J, and Israel Y. Identification of alcohol abuse using laboratory tests and a history of trauma. *Ann Intern Med* 1984; **101:** 847–51

6. Gill JS, Zezulda AV, Shipley MJ, Gill SK, and Beeevers DG. Stroke and alcohol consumption. *N Engl J Med* 1986; **315:** 1041–6

7. Holder HD and Blose JO. Alcoholism treatment and total health care utilization and costs. A four-year longitudinal analysis of federal employees. *JAMA* 1986; **256:** 1456–60

8. Reiff S, Griffiths B, Forsythe AB, and Sherman RM. Utilization of medical services by alcoholics participating in a health maintenance organization outpatient treatment program: three-year follow-up. *Alcohol Clin Exp Res* 1981; **5:** 559–62

9. Roghmann KJ, Roberts JS, Smith TS, Wells SM, and Wersinger RP. Alcoholics' versus nonalcoholics' use of services of a health maintenance organization. *J Stud Alcohol* 1981; **42:** 312–22

10. Klatsky AL, Friedman GD, and Siegelaub AB. Alcohol and mortality. A ten-year Kaiser-Permanente experience. *Ann Intern Med* 1981; **95:** 139–45

11. Moore RD, Bone LR, Geller G, Mamon JA, Stokes EJ, and Levine DM. Prevalence, detection, and treatment of alcoholism in hospitalized patients. *JAMA* 1989; **261:** 403–7

12. Beresford TP, Blow FC, Brower KJ, and Singer K. Screening for alcoholism. *Prev Med* 1988; **17:** 653–63

13. Ewing JA. Detecting alcoholism. The CAGE questionnaire. *JAMA* 1984; **252:** 1905–7

14. Mayfield D, McLeod G, and Hall P. The CAGE questionnaire: validation of a new alcoholism screening instrument. *Am J Psychiatry* 1974; **131:** 1121–3

15. Bush B, Shaw S, Cleary P, Delbanco TL, and Aronson MD. Screening for alcoholism using the CAGE questionnaire. *Am J Med* 1987; **82:** 231–5

16. King M. At risk drinking among general practice attenders: validation of the CAGE questionnaire. *Psychol Med* 1986; **16:** 213–7

17. Wallace P and Haines A. Use of a questionnaire in general practice to increase the recognition of patients with excessive alcohol consumption. *Br Med J* [*Clin Res*] 1985; **290:** 1949–53

18. Robinson KS, Burger MC, and Spickard WA. Tools for office diagnosis of alcoholism [Abstract]. *Clin Res* 1987; **35:** 92A

19. Ford DE and Kamerow DB. Screening for psychiatric and substance abuse disorders in clinical practice. *J Gen Intern Med* 1990; **5(Suppl 4):** S37–41

20. Robins LN, Helzer JE, Croughan J, and Ratcliff KS. National Institute of Mental Health Diagnostic Interview Schedule. Its history, characteristics, and validity. *Arch Gen Psychiatry* 1981; **38:** 381–9

21. American Psychiatric Association. Diagnostic and Statistical Manual of Mental Disorders. *Rev. 3d ed.* Washington, DC: American Psychiatric Association; 1987

22. Centor RM and Keightley GE. Receiver operating characteristics (ROC) curve area analysis using the ROC analyzer. Proceedings of the Thirteenth Annual Symposium on Computer Applications in Medical Care. Washington, DC, 5–8 November 1989

23. Hsiao JK, Bartko JJ, and Potter WZ. Diagnosing diagnoses. Receiver operating characteristic methods and psychiatry. *Arch Gen Psychiatry* 1989; **46**: 664–7

24. Gart JJ, and Nam J. Approximate interval estimation of the ratio of binomial parameters: a review and corrections for skewness. *Biometrics* 1988; **44**: 323–38

25. Koopman PA. Confidence intervals for the ratio of the two binomial proportions. *Biometrics* 1984; **40**: 513–7.

26. Pauker SG and Kassirer JP. The threshold approach to clinical decision making. *N Engl J Med* 1980; **302**: 1109–17

27. Fagan TJ. Nomogram for Baye's theorem [Letter]. *N Engl J Med* 1975; **293**: 257

28. Helzer JE, Spitznagel EL, and McEvoy L. The predictive validity of lay Diagnostic Interview Schedule diagnoses in the general population. *Arch Gen Psychiatry* 1987; **44**: 1069–77

29. Poses RM, Cebul RD, Collins M, and Fager SS. The importance of disease prevalence in transporting clinical prediction rules. The case of streptococcal pharyngitis. *Ann Intern Med* 1986; **105**: 586–91

30. Schwartz WB, Wolfe HJ, and Pauker SG. Pathology and probabilities: a new approach to interpreting and reporting biopsies. *N Engl J Med* 1981; **305**: 917–23

Complete the checklist

Now use the answers you have already given to complete the following checklist and assign a score to this paper. There is space for you to add comments about the paper before you decide your final score.

If you wish, you can compare your score and comments with ours, which you will find in the answers section at the back of the book. If you have access to the World Wide Web (via the Internet) you can also compare your scores with those of other readers of this book. Details of how to do this are given in Appendix III.

The checklist is designed to be generalized to other papers of this type. A full set of blank checklists is included at the end of the book, which can be copied for use with other papers.

RATING SCALE 2 FOR ARTICLE ON DIAGNOSIS/SCREENING

	Ring the appropriate code			
	Yes	Unclear/ possibly	No	Not applicable
RESULTS				
1 Are likelihood ratios (or necessary data) given?	2	1	0	N/A
2 Is the 'best cutpoint' of clinical importance?	2	1	0	N/A
(i.e. can the test usefully distinguish those with the disease from those without?)	2	1	0	N/A
3 Is the estimate of sensitivity/specificity (or likelihood ratio) sufficiently precise?	2	1	0	N/A
VALIDITY				
Selection				
4 Was the phase of the disease well defined?	2	1	0	N/A
5 Were patients at a uniform point in this phase?	2	1	0	N/A
6 Was the origin of the population of potential subjects (study population) described?	2	1	0	N/A
Measurement				
7 Was assessment against the gold standard 'blind'	2	1	0	N/A
8 Was the 'gold standard' applied to all subjects independent of the test result?	2	1	0	N/A
9 Could I repeat the study using the methods as described?	2	1	0	N/A
10 Was the repeatability of the test assessed?	2	1	0	N/A
Statistical analysis				
11 Were additional factors that might modify the test result (e.g. age, sex, disease phase) allowed for?	2	1	0	N/A
12 Were appropriate methods used?	2	1	0	N/A
13 Were any 'unusual' methods explained or justified?	2	1	0	N/A
(e.g. are methods easily found in a standard textbook – lots of references in MEDLINE? If so, it is probably not unusual)				
UTILITY				
14 For those who test positive do the results help me choose among alternative actions/treatments?	2	1	0	N/A
15 For those who test negative do the results help me reassure/counsel patients?	2	1	0	N/A

TOTAL (add ringed scores above):   _____ **(A)**

No. of questions which actually applied to this article (maximum = 15):   _____ **(B)**

Maximum possible score (2 × B):   _____ **(C)**

OVERALL RATING (A/C expressed as a percentage):   _____ %

COMMENTS:

EXERCISE 3 A paper on screening

LEARNING OBJECTIVES

After working through this exercise, you should be able to:

A Summarize and critically appraise a paper on screening for disease.

B Explain how the results in such a paper might apply to a clinical problem.

C Perform and interpret simple calculations found in such a paper.

KEY POINTS

- Algorithms can be a simple way to make use of multiple observations.

- The importance of misdiagnosis errors can be made explicit in a test.

- This approach could be generalized to patient symptoms and signs, investigations and other diseases.

CLINICAL RELEVANCE

- Is this screening test any use?

- Am I more concerned to avoid overdiagnosis or under-diagnosis?

THE CLINICAL PROBLEM

You are a resident medical officer working in a small rural mission hospital in Zimbabwe, about 200 km from the capital, Harare. You provide medical, surgical and obstetric services for the local population, and have a 'special care baby room' in the hospital where up to four babies can be cared for by a trained paediatric nurse.

Because of the poor maize harvest last year, you have found that in the last few months you have seen very many babies with low birth weights (LBW, meaning less than 2500 g). The special care room is always full.

As you start your daily ward round of the special care baby room, a message arrives from a village health worker. Three mothers in her village have given birth to LBW babies in the past 24 hours. Can she send them to you for special care?

As usual, the special care room is full, but the nurse feels that one baby is probably doing well enough to be moved out of the room, so you have one cot. You know you should use the cot for the least mature (lowest gestational age) baby, which is likely to be at higher risk of illness than babies which are more mature. Unfortunately, the village health worker says the mothers did not know their dates.

How can you help the village health worker to decide which baby needs the cot the most?

A POSSIBLE SOLUTION

Luckily, you are a member of an on-line library service. You switch on your laptop computer, dial into the library's MED-LINE database in London, and conduct a text search for 'screening', 'low birth weight' and 'preterm'. The search yields a single reference. After entering your credit card number, the system accepts your order for the reference you have found.

Two hours later, a copy of the paper arrives by fax.

You carefully read through the paper, hoping for help in deciding what to do. But how can you tell what the results mean? And is the paper relevant to your problem?

INTRODUCTION

Read the introduction to the paper, reproduced below, and answer the questions which follow it.

Low birthweight (LBW) and prematurity are important contributors to neonatal mortality and morbidity, especially in less developed countries, where these conditions are common.[1] Since few pregnant women in developing countries have prenatal care and most babies are born at home, ascertainment of birthweight and pregnancy duration is difficult. The baby's weight may not be measured for the first time until several days after birth, by which time substantial weight loss could have occurred. Widespread female illiteracy means that many women cannot record the dates of the last menstrual period or calculate duration of gestation. To overcome these difficulties, the usefulness of other neonatal body measurements, presumed to be more stable than birthweight, to identify LBW[2–13] or preterm[14] infants has been investigated. Such measurements include mid-arm, chest, and head circumferences.

No study so far has addressed the possibility that surrogate measurements could be used to classify babies by both gestational age and birthweight. In many developing countries, a large proportion of babies of LBW are delivered at term.[1,15] Because these infants are developmentally mature, their risk of neonatal mortality and morbidity is substantially lower than that of LBW babies born preterm.[16–19]

So that limited health care resources can be targeted at the highest-risk babies, a screening tool that reliably identifies only the subgroup of LBW babies who are also preterm would be very useful. We have developed an algorithm for this purpose that is both simple and accurate enough to be used by health workers outside the hospital setting.

---

1   Can you concisely express the research question to be addressed in this paper?

          _____

          _____

          _____

          _____

2   Explain why the authors consider it important to be able to identify preterm LBW infants separately from term LBW infants.

          _____

          _____

3   Why can LBW status not be determined simply by weighing the baby?

          _____

          _____

4   Suppose the researchers design a 'screening algorithm'. To be useful, what should the algorithm achieve?

          _____

          _____

5   In the context of a rural setting in a developing country, what features might you want to see in screening tests which are to be in widespread use?

          _____

          _____

          _____

          _____

METHODS

The next two sections of the paper describe the study subjects and measurements made on them.

Subjects

Data for the study were collected at the Tikur Anbessa Hospital, the primary referral centre serving the city of Addis Ababa, Ethiopia. The 5000 obstetric admissions per year consist of a mixture of high-risk referrals and self-referred low-risk patients. A transitional neonatal nursery and a special neonatal care unit adjoin the obstetric ward.

All infants admitted to the nursery or neonatal care unit between January, 1987, and December, 1988, were considered for the study. Of the total 1909, we excluded 1065 because of multiple birth (115), obvious congenital malformations (28), or uncertain gestational age (922). Gestational age was taken to be certain if the mother recalled the date of her last menstrual period, had had regular menses, and had not taken drugs known to affect ovulation, and if the gestational age calculated from the last menstrual period had been confirmed by clinical examination before 20 weeks' gestation. 1 infant admitted to the study was subsequently excluded from the analysis because the birthweight was miscoded at the time of data entry. Complete data were available for 843 infants.

Measurements

Gestational age was calculated from the first day of the last menstrual period. Maternal reports of menstrual history are reliable in this population because of cultural practices derived from Mosiac Laws and the special church calendar that permits dating of menses to within 1 or 2 days.[20] Birthweight was measured to the nearest 10 g on an infant beam balance scale within 24 h of birth. For this analysis, preterm was defined as birth before 259 days of gestation, and LBW as birthweight below 2500 g. High risk was defined as both preterm and LBW.

Measurements of neonatal chest, head, and mid-arm circumferences and length were obtained by trained paediatric nurse practitioners within 24 h of birth.[8, 13] The nurse practitioners were unaware of gestational age and birthweight measurements and of the study hypothesis.

6   Who were the subjects of the study?

_____

_____

7   Why were infants of uncertain gestational age excluded from the study population?

_____

_____

_____

_____

8   What measurements were collected for each of the babies in the study?

_____

_____

9   Why do you think the researchers made sure that the nurse practitioners who measured the babies were 'unaware of gestational age and birthweight'?

_____

_____

The remaining methods sections describe how the researchers generated their screening algorithms.

Misclassification costs

Because our aim was to develop a screening algorithm to be used to identify babies who might need referral for special paediatric care, we decided that false-negative errors (classifying a truly preterm, LBW baby as low risk) were more serious than false-positive errors (classifying a normal-weight or term baby as high risk). For the base-case analysis, the ratio of costs of these two misclassification errors, specified by a paediatrician (NT) with extensive experience in Africa, was taken as 10/1—i.e., misclassifying a preterm LBW baby as term or normal birthweight was ten times more serious than misclassifying a term or normal birthweight baby as preterm LBW. In the analysis and results, this relative cost was expressed by assigning arbitrary costs in penalty units to each type of misclassification error,[21] such that each false-positive error was assigned 1 unit, and each false-negative error 10 units. To investigate the effects of changing the specified cost ratio on the structure of our algorithm, we did a sensitivity analysis by regenerating the algorithm while varying the misclassification cost ratio from 1/1 to 50/1.

Development of algorithm

Since a predictive algorithm tends to be most accurate in the population from which it is derived, it is important to confirm its usefulness in an independent population.[22] We first divided the study population randomly in half to form training and validation groups. The training group was used to develop the screening algorithm. We expected that more than one of the four available surrogate neonatal measurements might be needed for the algorithm. To incorporate several measurements into the best screening strategy, we used a computerised statistical technique called recursive partitioning, which constructs a decision tree consisting of sequential binary decision nodes.[23]

First, the training group is divided into two subgroups, according to the value of the anthropometric measurement that would result in the lowest misclassification cost if the analysis ended there. Each subgroup is then partitioned again by another measurement with the same criterion. Partitioning is continued until little can be gained from further partitioning. Each terminal subset of the resulting classification tree is then assigned to the category (high or low risk) that generates the lowest overall misclassification cost. The tree is then 'pruned', to give a series of trees of decreasing complexity. For each tree in the series, the total misclassification cost and its standard error are estimated. The simplest tree with an estimated cost within one standard error of the lowest estimated cost is selected as the algorithm for the study.

Evaluation of algorithm

We calculated the sensitivity, specificity, and predictive accuracy of the selected algorithm to identify preterm, LBW babies as defined by recorded birthweight and gestational age. The average cost per patient was also calculated by dividing the sum of penalty units of all misclassification errors produced by the selected decision rule by the number of babies in the population.

10   The authors argue that, in using this test in a clinical setting, a false-negative error would be more serious than a false-positive error. Do you agree?

_____

_____

_____

_____

_____

11   To express the relative importance of these two possible errors (which any screening test can make), the authors use the idea of a 'misclassification cost ratio'. Explain, in plain language, what is implied by a misclassification cost ratio of:

a   50 : 1.

_____

_____

b   1 : 1.

_____

_____

c   1 : 10 (not considered in this paper).

_____

_____

12   What is a 'sensitivity analysis'?

_____

_____

_____

_____

_____

13   The study subjects were divided into two groups. What is the purpose of these groups?

_____

_____

_____

_____

_____

_____

The authors describe the technique of recursive partitioning, in which the computer generates a number of decision trees. Where trees are complex, they may be 'pruned' to simplify them.

14   How do the authors measure the performance of each tree that is generated?

_____

_____

_____

15   Are there any other criteria you might also want to consider in comparing various decision trees?

_____

_____

16   Explain, in plain language, how the 'best' tree is selected.

_____

_____

_____

_____

_____

RESULTS

The results section of this study is reproduced below. Read it carefully and answer the questions which follow.

Table 1 Comparison of training and validation groups

Mean (SD)	Training group (n = 422)	Validation group (n = 421)
Birthweight (g)	2952 (629)	2999 (544)
Gestational age (days)	276 (22·6)	277 (19·6)
Head circumference (cm)	34·5 (2·2)	34·7 (2·0)
Chest circumference (cm)	32·1 (3·0)	32·3 (2·6)
Mid-arm circumference (cm)	10·8 (1·3)	10·9 (1·1)
Length (cm)	48·8 (3·3)	49·1 (2·8)
Percentage of group		
LBW	17	13
Preterm	14	11
LBW and preterm	10	7

Algorithm A

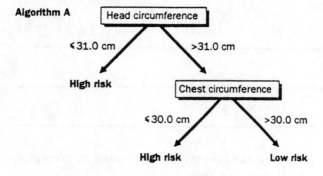

Algorithm B

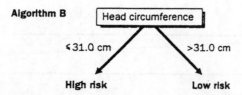

Figure Algorithms for distinguishing between high-risk (LBW and premature) and low-risk (normal-weight or full-term) infants.
Algorithm A used misclassification cost ratios ranging from 7·2/1 to 50/1, and algorithm B used ratios of 1/1 to 7·1/1.

There were no significant differences between the training and validation groups of babies in gestational age, birthweight, or other measurements (Student's t test, $p > 0·05$, 2-tailed) or in the proportions of LBW and preterm infants (Fisher's test, $p > 0·05$, 2-tailed, table 1). 70 of the 124 LBW babies in the study population were delivered before term.

The algorithm to distinguish between high-risk (LBW and premature) and low-risk (normal-weight or full-term) infants, with the initially specified misclassification cost ratio of 10/1, is given in the Figure (A). This algorithm required only two of the four measurements, head circumference and chest circumference. Infants with head circumferences of 31 cm or less or chest circumferences of 30 cm or less were classified as high risk. When tested in the validation group (Table 2), algorithm A had sensitivity, specificity, and negative predictive values above 90%. The positive predictive value was low (44%) because of the low prevalence of preterm, LBW babies in the population. The performance of the algorithm was nearly identical in the validation and training groups.

Table 2 Performance of base-case algorithm

	Training group (n = 422)	Validation group (n = 421)
Sensitivity (%)	95	93
Specificity (%)	92	92
Positive predictive value (%)	56	44
Negative predictive value (%)	99	99
Cost per patient (penalty units)	0·121	0·126

Table 3 Performance of algorithms generated with different misclassification cost ratios in validation group

	Algorithm B MCR = 1/1 to 7·1/1	Algorithm A MCR = 7·2/1 to 50/1
Sensitivity (%)	54	93
Specificity (%)	99	92
Positive predictive value (%)	83	44
Negative predictive value (%)	97	99

MCR = misclassification cost ratio.

The effect of changing the misclassification cost ratio on the structure of the algorithm was examined. The base-case algorithm (A) was generated throughout the range of cost ratios from 7·2/1 to 50/1. If a lower cost ratio was specified, however, the resulting algorithm was simpler, involving a single decision node of head circumference with a cutoff of 31 cm (Figure, B). Algorithm B, with the lower cost ratio, had lower sensitivity than algorithm A (Table 3), since the relative importance of missing a high-risk baby was lower; this algorithm also had higher specificity and positive predictive values.

17   What was the mean and standard deviation of the gestational age of babies in the training group?

18   What percentage of babies in each group were 'high risk'?

19   Examine Algorithm A given in the figure. Use it to allocate each of the babies in the table below to either a high risk or low risk category (write 'High' or 'Low' in column A). Then repeat the exercise with Algorithm B.

Subject	Head circumference (cm)	Chest circumference (cm)	Risk category using Algorithm A	Risk category using Algorithm B
Baby A	27	29		
Baby B	32	28		
Baby C	33	31		
Baby D	30	27		

20   Which subject(s) do the two algorithms classify differently?

_____

_____

_____

_____

21   Using Algorithm A, which babies could you still classify if you knew only:

a   The head circumference?

_____

b   The chest circumference?

_____

22   Explain why, if the assumed misclassification cost ratio falls from 10/1 to 1/1, the 'best tree' can be simplified from A to B.

_____

_____

_____

_____

23 Suppose we assume a misclassification cost ratio of 200/1. Explain what this would mean in reality, and how our assumption might alter the 'best tree' which results.

_____

_____

_____

_____

24 Examine Table 2, which shows how Algorithm A performs in each group of babies. You can see from the results presented that the algorithm has high sensitivity and specificity, but that the positive predictive value (PPV) is only around 50%. (See Box 3.1 for an explanation of these terms.)

a Explain what a PPV of 50% means in everyday terms.

_____

_____

_____

b Why is the PPV as low as this, despite the algorithm having high sensitivity and specificity?

_____

_____

_____

_____

DISCUSSION

The investigators' discussion is reproduced below. Read it carefully and answer the questions which follow.

This study shows that it is feasible to use neonatal body measurements to classify infants simultaneously by both gestational age and birthweight. Our algorithm was designed specifically to enable health-care workers in developing countries to screen for preterm, LBW infants. It requires two measurements, head and chest circumferences, and is simple enough to be easily learned and applied in field settings. When tested in an independent sample of babies, this algorithm showed sensitivity and specificity values both exceeding 90%.

Several potential limitations of our analysis should be addressed. First, the study population may not be representative of the general population of Ethiopia. Study subjects were recruited at a referral hospital, so the frequency of co-morbid conditions that affect body proportions might have been high. More than half the babies admitted to the hospital were ineligible for the study, mostly because of uncertain gestational age. Therefore, the validity of the algorithm elsewhere must be confirmed in future studies. Difficulties in obtaining accurate neonatal measurements in unselected populations are common to all studies of anthropometric neonatal screening tests in developing countries, and show the need for surrogate anthropometric screening tests in these settings.

Second, although it seems likely that the neonatal body measurements are stable after birth, this assumption has not, to our knowledge, been proven. A lack of stability would not affect the validity of the algorithm when used by traditional birth attendants or other health workers present at delivery, but it might limit the usefulness for infants not seen until several days after birth. To resolve this issue, longitudinal studies of neonatal measurements in less developed settings will be required.

Finally, gestational age was calculated in this study from reported last menstrual period, and was not confirmed by ultrasound. Although we took care to ensure that only women with reliable menstrual histories confirmed by early obstetric examination were included, some inaccuracy in gestational dating is possible.

Our study differs from previous studies of neonatal anthropometric screening tools[2-14] in several respects. First, we defined high-risk babies as being both preterm and LBW. We chose this definition to enhance the public health usefulness of the algorithm, by excluding the large proportion of LBW babies in developing countries who are born at term[1,15] and who therefore have a lower risk of neoatal mortality and morbidity.[18] Classification of babies by both gestational age and birthweight should be possible with a combination of body measurements because of the differences in body proportions between preterm and growth-retarded term LBW infants. Normally grown preterm babies tend to have larger bodies in relation to head size than growth-retarded babies of the same birthweight.[24] Although this disproportionality among growth-retarded babies may be less common in developing than in developed countries,[25] it is interesting that our base-case algorithm included both head circumference and a measure of body size (chest circumference).

Unlike previous studies, our analysis was specifically designed to create an algorithm that kept to a minimum the clinical impact of misclassification errors in the population. For any predictive algorithm, the relative importance of false-negative and false-positive diagnoses depends on the intended application.[22] In the clinical setting for which our algorithm was developed, identifying a truly high-risk baby as low-risk would certainly be more serious than the reverse error. By contrast, in a research setting where the goal is to define the prevalence of a high-risk and low-risk babies, false-positive and false-negative errors might be judged equally unacceptable, and thus a relative cost ratio of 1/1 would be more appropriate. The effect of the choice of cost ratio is shown by our sensitivity analysis. The algorithm derived with the higher ratio had substantially higher sensitivity, consistent with its intended application as a clinical screening tool.

The statistical method used in this study, recursive partitioning, has not been used in previous attempts to devise neonatal anthropometric screening tools. This method is well suited to the construction of clinical screening instruments that include several predictive variables. It generates algorithms that incorporate only one observation at a time and that directly define distinct clusters of high-risk and low-risk patients without the need for calculations or special equipment, which limit the use of screening tools developed with other multivariate techniques.[5,12] In addition, because of their hierarchical nature, algorithms created by recursive partitioning can allow classification of subjects without complete information. For example, in our base-case algorithm, a baby whose head circumference was less than 31 cm could be classified as high risk without the need for chest measurement. Recursive partitioning is also quite robust—extreme outliers do not have a great effect on the structure of the final selected algorithm. This robustness partly explains why there was little difference in the performance of the base-case algorithm in the training and validation groups in this study and may imply that the algorithm is applicable to new populations with less loss of sensitivity and specificity than screening tools created by other multivariate techniques such as logistic regression.

In future studies, the algorithm proposed here should be adapted and revalidated for use in specific populations. Ultimately, the value of this screening tool must be judged by its ability to improve neonatal health when incorporated into a coordinated system of primary health care, referral, and treatment.

Box 3.1: What makes a good screening test?

The purpose of a screening test is to separate, as far as is possible, those individuals who do have a particular condition from those who do not. There are a number of ways in which the ability of a test to do this can be expressed.

The **sensitivity** of a test is a measure of its ability to detect cases of a condition. It is defined as:

Sensitivity = (subjects with condition correctly detected by test)/
            (all subjects with condition)

The **specificity** of a test is a measure of its ability not to give a positive result when the condition is absent. It is defined as:

Specificity = (subjects without condition correctly detected by test)/
            (all subjects without condition)

Both the sensitivity and specificity measure the ability of the test to come to correct conclusions about individuals. For both, the higher the value, the better.

Neither of these measures is of great interest to the individual patient who has just received a positive test result, however. For such a person, or their doctor, the important question is: given that I have a positive result, what are the chances that I have the condition? This question is answered by the **positive predictive value**, defined as:

Positive predictive value = (subjects who actually have the condition)/
            (all subjects who test positive).

In many situations it is important that people are not alarmed unnecessarily by a positive test result when they do not, in fact, have the condition. A high positive predictive value is therefore desirable.

Similarly, the **negative predictive value** is defined as the proportion of those who test negative who do not, in fact, have the condition.

Of course, having good performance characteristics is not enough to ensure a test can be used in practice. A good test should also be:

- Acceptable to individuals – not embarrassing, painful or harmful.
- Quick and easy to perform and interpret.
- Inexpensive.

Where to find out more

Donaldson RJ and Donaldson LJ. *Essential Public Health Medicine.* Kluwer Academic, Lancaster, 1993

25   What are the three potential limitations to which the authors draw attention?

_____

_____

_____

Box 3.2: What makes a good screening programme?

A new screening programme for a given condition in a given population cannot, of course, be introduced without a suitable screening test (see Box 3.1). However, the existence of a sensitive, specific, cheap and acceptable test is not, in itself, sufficient to ensure that a proposed programme of screening is likely to do more good than harm to a population's health.

The most important single criterion, and one which is surprisingly often overlooked, is that *there must be good evidence that earlier recognition of the condition can result in a better outcome for the individual*. It is implicit in this criterion that there is a course of action which can be taken (usually earlier treatment) which improves outcome. If evidence that early action can improve outcome does not exist, it would be hard to support the introduction of a full-scale programme of screening, but a limited, pilot programme might be justified in order to gather the evidence that is required.

Given a suitable test and good evidence that early diagnosis can be beneficial, there are a number of important questions which should be asked about the organizational aspects of a screening programme before it goes ahead:

Is the population to be screened clearly defined? Is it clear who should be invited for screening and who should not?

How will the target population be invited for screening (and re-screening)? A system for inviting people for screening must ensure that the whole target population is covered, and that people can be recalled for rescreening or further investigation easily.

Is there an agreed definition of 'cases' and an agreed policy for 'borderline' results? It is important that any given test result can lead to an unambiguous response.

Are there adequate facilities for the investigation and treatment of 'cases'? Any new screening programme is likely to lead to a large number of extra diagnostic tests and some extra treatment being required, all of which need resources to be available (not just of money, but also possibly buildings, equipment, trained personnel, etc.).

Will there be a system for monitoring the effectiveness of the programme? Information should be collected both on how the programme is running and on the outcomes, such as disease mortality, which the programme aims to improve.

Is the programme likely to be cost-effective in comparison with other ways of gaining similar benefits? An economic evaluation should be done to indicate the likely costs and benefits of the programme. It may be that other approaches to the problem, such as primary prevention, or improving treatment facilities, would be a better use of resources.

Where to find out more

Donaldson RJ and Donaldson LJ. *Essential Public Health Medicine*. Kluwer Academic, Lancaster, 1993

Box 3.3: Evaluation of a screening programme

If a new screening programme met all the requirements set out in Boxes 3.1 and 3.2, we would be confident that, in principle, it would be likely to lead to health benefits – such as improved cancer survival – in a screened population. However, we could not be sure that such benefits had been achieved until we evaluated the programme in the real world. Such an evaluation should examine both how the programme runs – process evaluation – and the health impact of the programme on the population – outcome evaluation.

A good **process** evaluation should look at measures which give an indication of the organizational quality and efficiency of the programme. Such measures might include the proportion of the invited population which is screened, the speed of test reporting, the time a person with a positive result must wait before having a definitive investigation, or the proportion of people with positive results who turn out not to have the condition. The latter is *also* sometimes termed the false-positive rate, a different definition from that used in Box 2.3.

The evaluation of screening programme **outcomes** is not so straightforward. Although the aim of a screening test, for example for cancer, is improved survival, simply showing that screened individuals have a longer survival time than non-screened individuals is inadequate to establish the effectiveness of the programme. Such an observation may be influenced by three potential biases, as follows:

Lead time bias: If screening leads to a disease being diagnosed earlier than it otherwise would have been, then the *apparent* survival (the time between diagnosis and death) will be increased by virtue of this fact alone, whether or not death can be delayed. This apparently extra survival time (the time between diagnosis on screening and when diagnosis would occur without screening) is termed lead time, and must be taken into account in an evaluation.

Length bias: Not all cases of a given disease progress at the same rate. Individuals with slowly progressing disease are likely to be over-represented among screen-detected cases, compared to those with rapidly progressing disease, who are not in a pre-symptomatic stage long enough to be detected by screening. However, those with slowly progressing disease are also likely to have the better prognosis, leading to the observation that screen-detected cases have a better prognosis than non-screen detected cases – not because people benefit from the screening, but because screening picks out those people who will do better anyway. This is a form of selection bias.

Self-selection bias (see also Box 4.3): A further kind of selection bias may occur if, as is often the case, those who attend for screening are also those who would have a better prognosis if they developed the disease. This may occur if those who attend tend to be younger, more educated or more wealthy than those who do not, since all of these factors may in themselves be associated with improved outcome.

In assessing the outcomes of screening, a study must take into account all of these possibilities.

Where to find out more

Hennekens CH and Buring JE. *Epidemiology in Medicine.* Little, Brown and Co, Boston, 1987

26   Given the measurements which were collected, what alternative approaches to developing a screening test might have been tried? What are the advantages and disadvantages of the recursive partitioning method used here?

_____

_____

_____

_____

_____

_____

_____

_____

_____

_____

_____

_____

_____

_____

_____

_____

_____

_____

27 Do you agree with the authors' main conclusion that 'it is feasible to use neonatal body measurements to classify infants simultaneously by both gestational age and birthweight'?

_____

Does the paper help you with your problem?

28 Now return to the clinical problem you started with. What factors would you want to consider in deciding whether the findings of the paper apply in your situation?

_____

_____

_____

_____

_____

29 Has this paper helped you to solve your problem?

_____

_____

_____

_____

_____

_____

Finally, here is the authors' summary of the paper.

SUMMARY

Preterm, low-birthweight (LBW) newborn infants are at high risk of neonatal mortality and morbidity and need early referral for special paediatric care. In developing countries, birthweight and gestational age often cannot be measured and a practical screening tool based on surrogate neonatal body measurements to identify high-risk infants would be very useful. We studied a consecutive series of 843 singleton infants born at a referral hospital in Addis Ababa, Ethiopia. Gestational age, birthweight, and four body measurements (chest, head, and mid-arm circumferences and length) were accurately recorded. We randomly divided the series into equal-sized training and validation groups. In the training group, we used a recursive partitioning technique to develop a simple predictive algorithm—infants were classified as high risk if head circumference was 31 cm or less or if chest circumference was 30 cm or less, and were classified as low risk otherwise. When tested in the validation group, this algorithm had sensitivity, specificity, and negative predictive value for prediction of preterm and LBW births above 90%. Thus, neonatal body measurements can be combined into a pragmatic, accurate screening tool suitable for clinical use in developing countries.

30 Is the summary a fair reflection of the evidence presented?

_____

_____

_____

Title

Development of a practical screening tool to identify preterm, low-birthweight neonates in Ethiopia Elizabeth G Raymond, Nebiat Tafari, James F Troendle, John D Clemens

Lancet 1994; **344:** 520–23

Division of Epidemiology, Statistics, and Prevention Research, National Institute of Child Health and Human Development, National Institutes of Health, Building 6100, Room 7B03, Rockville, MD 20852, USA (E G Raymond MD, N Tafari MD, J F Troendle PhD, J D Clemens MD), and Department of Pediatrics, Faculty of Medicine, Addis Ababa University, Addis Ababa, Ethiopia (N Tafari).

Correspondence to: Dr John D Clemens.

References

1. Villar J and Belizan J. The relative contribution of prematurity and fetal growth retardation to low birth weight in developing and developed societies. _Am J Obstet Gynecol_ 1982; **143:** 793–98

2. Alves JGB, Lima GMDS, Azevedo GNDA, Cabral VBC, Moggi RS, and Nunes R. Evaluation of newborn arm circumference as an indicator of low birth weight. _Bull Pan Am Health Organ_ 1991; **25:** 207–09

3. Bhargava SK, Ramji S, Kumar A, Mohan M, Marwah J, and Sachdev HPS. Mid-arm and chest circumferences at birth as predictors of low birth weight and neonatal mortality in the community. _BMJ_ 1985; **291:** 1617–19

4. Diamond ID, Abd El-Aleem AM, Ali MY, Mostafa SAM, El-Nashar SMA, and Giudotti RJ. The relationship between birth weight and arm and chest circumference in Egypt. _J Trop Pediatr_ 1991; **37:** 323–26

5. Dusitsin N, Chompootaweep S, Poomsuwan P, Susitsin K, Sentrakul P, and Lumbiganond P. Development and validation of a simple device to estimate birthweight and screen for low birthweight in developing countries. _Am J Public Health_ 1991; **81:** 1201–05

6. Gozal D, Ndombo PK, Minkande JZ, Kago I, Tetanye E, and Mbede J. Anthropometric measurements in a newborn population in West Africa: a reliable and simple tool for the identification of infants at risk for early postnatal morbidity. _J Pediatr_ 1991; **118:** 800–05

7. Huque F and Hussain AMZ. Detection of low birth-weight new born babies by anthropometric measurements in Bangladesh. _Indian J Pediatr_ 1991; **58:** 223–31

8. Landicho B, Lechtig A, and Klein RE. Anthropometric indicators of low birth weight. _J Trop Pediatr_ 1985; **31:** 301–05

9. Mohan M, Chellani HK, Prasad SRS, and Kapani V. Intrauterine growth predictors. *Indian Pediatr* 1991; **28**: 1299–304

10. Neela J, Raman L, Balakrishna N, and Rao KV. Usefulness of calf circumference as a measure for screening low birth weight infants. *Indian Pediatr* 1991; **28**: 881–84

11. Sauerborn R, Ouiminga RM, Kone B, Sama R, Oepen C, and Ebrahim GJ. Neonatal mid-upper-arm circumference is a valid proxy for birth weight. *Trop Med Parasitol* 1990; **41**: 65–67

12. Sharma JN, Saxena S, and Sharma U. Ratio of mid arm circumference to head circumference as a predictor of small for gestational age babies. *Indian J Pediatr* 1989; **26**: 348–50

13. World Health Organization Collaborative study of Birth Weight Surrogates. Use of a simple anthropometric measurement to predict birth weight. *Bull World Health Organ* 1993; **71**: 157–63

14. Eregie CO. Assessment of gestational age: the value of a maturity scoring system for head circumference and mid-arm circumference. *J Trop Pediatr* 1991; **37**: 182–84

15. Villar J, Khoury MJ, Finucane FF, and Delgado HL. Differences in the epidemiology of prematurity and intrauterine growth retardation. *Early Hum Dev* 1986; **14**: 307–20

16. Arias F and Tomich P. Etiology and outcome of low birth weight and preterm infants. *Obstet Gynecol* 1982; **60**: 277–81

17. Starfield B, Shapiro S, McCormick M, and Bross D. Mortality and morbidity in infants with intrauterine growth retardation. *J Pediatr* 1982; **101**: 978–93

18. Victora CG, Barros FC, Vaughan JP, and Teixeira AMB. Birthweight and infant mortality: a longitudinal study of 5914 Brazilian children. *Int J Epidemiol* 1987; **16**: 239–45

19. Gray RH, Ferraz EM, Amorim MS, and DeMelo LF. Levels and determinants of early neonatal mortality in Natal, Northeastern Brazil: results of a surveillance and case control study. *Int J Epidemiol* 1991; **20**: 467–73

20. Gebre-Medhin M, Sterky G, and Taube A. Observations on intrauterine growth in urban Ethiopia. *Acta Paediatr Scand* 1978; **67**: 781–89

21. Goldman L, Weinberg M, Weisberg M, et al. A computer-derived protocol to aid in the diagnosis of emergency room patients with acute chest pain. *N Engl J Med* 1982; **307**: 588–96

22. Wasson JH, Sox HC, Neff RK, and Goldman L. Clinical prediction rules: applications and methodological standards. *N Engl J Med* 1985; **313**: 793–99

23. Breiman L, Friedman JH, Olshen RA, and Stone CJ. Classification and regression trees. Monterey CA: Wadsworth and Brooks, 1984

24. Kramer MS, McLean FH, Olivier M, Willis DM, and Usher RH. Body proportionality and head and length 'sparing' in growth retarded neonates: a critical reappraisal *Pediatrics* 1989; **84**: 717–23

25. Villar J, Altobelli L, Kestler E, and Belizan J. A health priority for developing countries: the prevention of chronic fetal malnutrition. *Bull World Health Organ* 1986; **64**: 847–51

Complete the checklist

Now use the answers you have already given to complete the following checklist and assign a score to this paper. There is space for you to add comments about the paper before you decide your final score.

If you wish, you can compare your score and comments with ours, which you will find in the answers section at the back of the book. If you have access to the World Wide Web (via the Internet) you can also compare your scores with those of other readers of this book. Details of how to do this are given in Appendix III.

The checklist is designed to be generalized to other papers of this type. A full set of blank checklists is included at the end of the book, which can be copied for use with other papers.

RATING SCALE 2 FOR ARTICLE ON DIAGNOSIS/SCREENING

		Ring the appropriate code			
		Yes	Unclear/ possibly	No	Not applicable
RESULTS					
1	Are likelihood ratios (or necessary data) given?	2	1	0	N/A
2	Is the 'best cutpoint' of clinical importance?	2	1	0	N/A
	(i.e. can the test usefully distinguish those with the disease from those without?)	2	1	0	N/A
3	Is the estimate of sensitivity/specificity (or likelihood ratio) sufficiently precise?	2	1	0	N/A
VALIDITY					
Selection					
4	Was the phase of the disease well defined?	2	1	0	N/A
5	Were patients at a uniform point in this phase?	2	1	0	N/A
6	Was the origin of the population of potential subjects (study population) described?	2	1	0	N/A
Measurement					
7	Was assessment against the gold standard 'blind'	2	1	0	N/A
8	Was the 'gold standard' applied to all subjects independent of the test result?	2	1	0	N/A
9	Could I repeat the study using the methods as described?	2	1	0	N/A
10	Was the repeatability of the test assessed?	2	1	0	N/A
Statistical analysis					
11	Were additional factors that might modify the test result (e.g. age, sex, disease phase) allowed for?	2	1	0	N/A
12	Were appropriate methods used?	2	1	0	N/A
13	Were any 'unusual' methods explained or justified? (e.g. are methods easily found in a standard textbook – lots of references in MEDLINE? If so, it is probably not unusual)	2	1	0	N/A
UTILITY					
14	For those who test positive do the results help me choose among alternative actions/treatments?	2	1	0	N/A
15	For those who test negative do the results help me reassure/ counsel patients?	2	1	0	N/A

TOTAL (add ringed scores above): _____ **(A)**

No. of questions which actually applied to this article (maximum = 15): _____ **(B)**

Maximum possible score (2 × B): _____ **(C)**

OVERALL RATING (A/C expressed as a percentage): _____ %

COMMENTS:

EXERCISE 4 A paper on causation of disease

LEARNING OBJECTIVES

After working through this exercise, you should be able to:

A Summarize and critically appraise a paper on causation of a disease.

B Explain how the results in such a paper might apply to a clinical problem.

C Perform and interpret simple calculations found in such a paper.

KEY POINTS

- It is not ethical to subject individuals to potentially harmful exposures.

- Studies of disease causation must therefore be observational.

- Studies compare groups of individuals either according to their exposure status or disease status.

- An association between exposure and outcome does not prove causation.

CLINICAL RELEVANCE

- How can I advise patients to stay healthy?

- Does this treatment carry any risks?

THE CLINICAL PROBLEM

You are a general practitioner. One night you are telephoned at 10 p.m. by a distraught mother of four who is at the local hospital. Her eldest daughter, aged 22 years, had collapsed at home and was rushed to the accident and emergency department by ambulance. Tragically, by the time the ambulance reached the hospital her daughter had died. The casualty consultant has said something about a 'clot on the lung'.

You agree to visit the family the following morning. You call in at your surgery to pick up the daughter's case notes, and notice that she had recently been started on the oral contraceptive pill by one of your partners.

Could this have contributed in any way to her untimely death? What should you say to the family?

A POSSIBLE SOLUTION

In order to get some up-to-date information, you quickly search the practice's MEDLINE CD-ROM for recent studies of thromboembolism and oral contraceptive use. Your search yields a handful of studies. Fortunately, one of these is immediately available on the shelves of the practice library. You go to the library, find the paper, and read it through.

INTRODUCTION

Read the introduction to the paper, reproduced below, and answer the questions which follow it.

An increased risk of venous thromboembolism in association with oral contraceptive use was first identified in a case-control study in 1967.[1] The association has been confirmed many times subsequently, both in case-control and cohort studies, with the estimated increase in risk ranging between 2- and 11-fold.[2] There is evidence from several epidemiological studies that the level of increased risk is associated with the dose of oestrogen in the contraceptive preparation,[2] and this finding has been supported in clinical studies of the effects of oral contraceptive preparations on haemostatic variables.[3,4] There is also some evidence that the type of progestogen used can affect the coagulation system.[5]

In recent years, the formulation of oral contraceptive preparations in common use has been changing, with a trend towards lower doses of both oestrogen and progestogen.[6] We have therefore re-examined the association between oral contraceptive use and fatal venous thromboembolism.

1   In one sentence, identify the question which this study aims to answer, in terms of patient type, exposure and outcome.

_____

_____

_____

_____

2   The authors say this issue has been studied 'many times' in the past. Why do they feel it should be re-investigated now?

_____

_____

_____

_____

3   Briefly outline how you might go about investigating this research question. What approaches might you consider?

_____

_____

_____

_____

_____

_____

_____

_____

_____

_____

_____

METHODS

The next section of the paper describes what the investigators did. Read it, and answer the questions which follow.

Identification of cases

The study described here formed part of a larger study of mortality from cardiovascular disease, including myocardial infarction and stroke, as well as venous thromboembolism. The methodology of the study has been described in detail previously.[7] Briefly, in this part of the study all deaths occurring in England and Wales among women aged 16–39 between January 1986 and December 1988 where the underlying cause of death was coded as pulmonary embolism (ICD-9 415·1), or venous thromboembolism (ICD-9 451–453) were considered for inclusion. Cases were excluded if there was insufficient evidence to confirm the cause of death, if the woman had been resident for at least one month in an institution, or if she had been pregnant within the last two months before death. Deaths that were preceded by another life threatening illness such as advanced cancer were also excluded.

Selection of controls and collection of clinical data

The general practitioner of each case was identified and interviewed using a structured questionnaire, by a part-time medical officer employed by the Committee on Safety of Medicines. Two control women, matched for age (within 5-year groups) and marital status (two categories: currently married or living as married, or not) were selected randomly from the practice records of the same general practitioner. The same criteria for exclusion were applied as for the cases, and a similar questionnaire was completed for the control women. In a few cases, controls were excluded at the analysis stage because they fell within the exclusion criteria (e.g. controls who appeared by backward calculation to have been pregnant at the time of death of the relevant matched case). The identity of the control women was not recorded on the completed questionnaires in the interests of confidentiality.

The general practitioners were asked for details of past medical history, (including any diagnosis of cardiovascular disease or hypertension or any other major illness) drug history, (particularly use of oral contraceptives), menstrual status, obstetric history, contraceptive methods, parity, height, weight, blood pressure and smoking habits.

Postal questionnaire data

An attempt was made to collect additional information concerning smoking habits from postal questionnaires if the case was married or living as married and the general practitioner knew the whereabouts of the surviving partner. A brief questionnaire was sent both to the surviving partner and to the corresponding pair of control women. Unfortunately, only 20 such case-control sets were identified, and only five questionnaires were returned by surviving partners, and, accordingly, data from the postal questionnaires have not been included in the analysis.

Analysis

Oral contraceptive use was assigned to one of three categories: use in the month before death (or the corresponding time for the controls), described in this paper as current use; use in the preceding ten years but not in the last month, described in this paper as previous use; and no use within ten years (including women who had never used oral contraceptives), described in this paper as non-use.

Data were entered on a personal computer using Dbase, and then transferred to the University of Oxford VAX cluster. Simple two- and three-way tables were constructed and statistical significance was tested by χ^2 test, or, where appropriate, by Fisher's exact test using the statistical package SPSSX. Statistical significance was reported if $P < 0.05$. Odds ratios (OR) were estimated by conditional logistic regression analysis adjusting for the effects of matching[8] using the computer software EGRET[9] to estimate odds ratios. The estimated OR and 95% confidence intervals are reported. All estimations are based on 60 matched case-control sets (including any sets that were concordant in outcome for a particular variable). The power of the study was estimated using the computer software EPILOG POWER.[10]

4   What type of study design have the authors chosen? Briefly outline the important features of this design.

_____

_____

_____

_____

_____

5   Do you think this choice of study design was appropriate in this instance?

_____

_____

_____

_____

_____

6   How were the cases identified? Is the diagnosis of cases well defined?

_____

_____

_____

_____

7   How were controls identified? Are the controls drawn from 'the same population' as the cases?

_____

_____

_____

_____

8   What information was collected about each study subject?

_____

_____

_____

_____

9   The researchers 'matched cases and controls with respect to age and marital status'. What was the purpose of doing this?

_____

_____

_____

10   List the reasons why some women were excluded from the study.

_____

_____

11   Why did the investigators exclude these potential subjects?

_____

_____

_____

12   How was exposure to the oral contraceptive pill measured in this study? Would you expect this method to be accurate and free from bias?

_____

_____

_____

_____

_____

_____

_____

RESULTS

Table 1 shows the number of cases of fatal venous thromboembolism considered for entry into the study, together with the reasons for exclusion. There were 67 cases that were eligible for inclusion, seven (10%) were excluded for administrative reasons. Amongst the 60 cases that were included there were 14 cases where the cause of death was given as pulmonary embolism without mention of a venous thrombosis, and 46 cases where the cause was given as venous thrombosis. Cause of death was confirmed by the finding of thrombus or embolus at dissection of the veins or lungs post mortem in 54 cases (90%). In the remaining six cases, the diagnosis was confirmed by venogram or lung scan antemortem. Of the cases 26 (44%) were aged under 25 years, 16 (27%) were aged between 25 and 34 years, and 18 (30%) were aged 35–39 years. There were 115 matched control women. The date of birth of three controls was not completed on the questionnaire, although it is known that they were age matched to the cases as instructed. Four controls (3%), were aged 40, but were included in the analysis. Of the controls 46 (40%) were aged under 25 years, 38 controls (33%) were aged 25 to 34 years, and 24 controls (21%) were aged 35–39 years.

Five cases (8%) had a history of previous deep vein thrombosis and four (7%) a history of superficial vein thrombosis. None of the controls had a history of either of these conditions. There were also four cases (7%) and one control (1%) with a history of previous pulmonary embolism. The estimated OR of fatal venous thromboembolism associated with a history of any previous venous thrombotic episode was 4·0 (95% CI: 1·4–11·5).

General practitioners were asked whether the women had undergone an operation or been involved in an accident within the three months prior to the death of the case. Seven cases (12%) and three controls (3%) had had such an experience. The estimated OR of fatal venous thromboembolism associated with surgery or an accident within 3 months was 11·1 (95% CI: 1·3–92·5).

There were no significant differences between the cases and controls in the frequency of any one of the other diseases specifically listed on the questionnaire (hypertension, stroke, diabetes, hyperlipidaemia or heart disease). However, the questionnaire also included a general question about 'any other major illness of relevance'. There were 29 cases (48%) and 19 controls (17%) who were reported to have had such an illness. This difference was highly significant in an unmatched analysis ($P < 0.001$). Overall, 40 (67%) cases and 29 (25%) controls were reported to have had at least one previous major diagnosis (including all the specific diagnoses listed on the questionnaire as well as the other major illnesses mentioned).

The records of each of the cases and controls who were reported to have had a 'major illness of relevance' were examined individually. Five cases, but none of the controls were reported to be mentally retarded ($P < 0.01$, Fisher's exact test, not adjusted for matching), four cases but no controls had a history of epilepsy ($P < 0.05$ Fisher's exact test, not adjusted for matching). No other

Table 1 Death certificates received, numbers considered for entry into the study, and reasons for exclusion

Certificates received	91
Reasons for exclusion:	
Woman not resident in England and Wales	2
Pregnant or within 2 months post-partum	13
Resident in an institution	3
Already gravely ill with cancer, renal failure or neurological disease	1
Diagnosis not confirmed	5
Considered for entry into the study	67
Medical notes lost	2
General practitioner not traced	3
PTMO unable to obtain interview with GP	2
Total included	60
	(90% of those considered)

differences were statistically significant and neither of these diagnoses had an estimated OR adjusted for the effects of matching with a lower confidence limit above 1. Moreover, the importance of these differences should not be overemphasized, since they were not specifically enquired about, and it may well be that the general practitioners would have volunteered a greater amount of additional information about women who had died than about living controls.

Of the 38 cases for whom smoking information was available in the general practice notes, 11 (29%) were current smokers. There were 58 controls for whom this information was available, and 23 (40%) were current smokers. This difference was not significant.

Table 2 shows the overall use of oral contraceptives amongst cases and controls. Exclusion of those women who had undergone surgical sterilization resulted in very little change. There was, however, a very substantial amount of morbidity amongst the cases, and many of the thrombotic events could not be described as clearly 'idiopathic'. Table 3 shows the oral contraceptive use of cases and controls according to three different categories of exclusions used to define idiopathic cases. The Table first shows use excluding those women who had had an operation or experienced an accident in the last three months, then, secondly, excluding in addition women with a previous history of venous thromboembolism or other blood vessel or heart disease, at any time. Finally, the third analysis excludes all these women and, in addition, women who had severely limited mobility, and women who had a diagnosis of haemoglobinopathy or other blood disorder. None of the differences between cases and controls in use of oral contraceptives was significant.

The overall estimated OR of fatal venous thromboembolism associated with current use of oral contraceptives was 1·6 (95% CI: 0·7–3·4). After controlling for the presence of other conditions, (i.e. all the conditions listed as exclusions in Table 3), the estimated OR rose to 2·1 (95% CI: 0·8–5·2). Of the 26 cases who were currently using oral contraceptives, 15 were using combined preparations with 35 µg or less of oestrogen, one was using a combined preparation with 50 µg of oestrogen, 10 were using multiphasic preparations, and the preparation used by three cases was unknown. The equivalent numbers for the 45 control women who were current users were 24, 2, 17, and 2. None of the women in this study was using progestogen only preparations.

Seven cases and three controls had had an accident or operation in the 3 months preceding the death. Of these ten women, four of the cases, but none of the controls, were currently using oral contraceptives.

Table 2 Oral contraceptive use in cases and controls (percentages in parentheses)

Oral contraceptive use	Cases	Controls
All women		
Nonusers	20 (33)	39 (34)
Previous users	11 (18)	31 (27)
Current users	29 (48)	45 (39)
Total	60 (100)	115 (100)

13 The study shows an association between fatal thromboembolism and a previous venous thrombotic episode. Explain, in plain language, the meaning of the odds ratio (OR) and its confidence interval (CI).

_____

_____

_____

_____

_____

Box 4.1: Relative risk, odds and odds ratios

If we do a typical cohort study, we follow up subjects from the time of exposure to see what proportions become ill in the 'exposed' and 'unexposed' groups. The data can be laid out as follows, where the letters a, b, c and d denote the number of subjects who end up in each category:

	Become ill	Do not	Total
Exposed	a	b	a + b
Unexposed	c	d	c + d

The risk of disease in the exposed group is: $a/(a + b)$ while the risk in the unexposed group is $c/(c + d)$.

The relative risk (RR), or risk ratio, is simply the risk in those exposed divided by the risk in those unexposed:

$$RR = \{a/(a + b)\}/\{c/(c + d)\}$$

If the disease is rare, even in the exposed group a will be much smaller than $(a + b)$, so that $(a + b)$ will approximately equal b; likewise in the unexposed group $(c + d)$ will approximately equal d, so that the relative risk is approximately:

$$RR \approx \{a/b\}/\{c/d\} = ad/bc$$

Another way of looking at risk is in terms of odds (see Box 2.1). By definition if the *risk* is the probability of something, denoted by p, then the *odds* of the event are:

$$Odds = P/(1 - P) \approx P, \text{ if the risk is very small so that } 1 - P \approx 1$$

The approximate relative risk found above is, in fact, precisely the odds ratio of disease given exposure (i.e. odds of disease if exposed, divided by odds of disease if unexposed).

In contrast to cohort studies, case-control studies compare (strictly speaking) the exposure of cases with that of controls:

	Cases	Controls
Exposed	a	b
Unexposed	c	d
Total	(a + c)	(b + d)

But we need not compare the proportion of cases exposed with the proportion of controls exposed. We can look at the *odds of exposure* in the two groups instead:

Odds of exposure for cases = a/c

Odds of exposure for controls = b/d

The ratio of these values is ad/bc, and this is the *same* as the odds ratio from a cohort study that approximates the relative risk.

So, if the outcome is rare, the odds ratio (OR) from a case-control study approximates the relative risk (RR) that we would have obtained, had we been able to do a cohort study in the first place.

Where to find out more

Hennekens CH and Buring JE. *Epidemiology in Medicine.* Little, Brown and Co, Boston, 1987; pp 77–82

Table 3 Oral contraceptive use in cases and controls excluding women with morbidity (percentages in parentheses)

Oral contraceptive use	Cases	Controls
Excluding women with an operation or accident in last 3 months		
Nonusers	18 (34)	39 (35)
Previous users	10 (19)	28 (25)
Current users	25 (47)	45 (40)
Total	53 (100)	112 (100)
Also excluding women with any history of venous thromboembolism or other blood vessel or heart disease		
Nonusers	15 (34)	36 (34)
Previous users	7 (16)	26 (25)
Current users	22 (50)	44 (42)
Total	44 (100)	106 (100)
Also excluding women with limited mobility or a diagnosis of haemoglobinopathy or other blood disorder		
Nonusers	1? (29)	34 (33)
Previous users	7 (17)	25 (24)
Current users	22 (54)	44 (43)
Total	41 (100)	103 (100)

14 An association is also apparent with a history of recent operation or accident. What reservations might you have about accepting this result at face value?

_____

_____

_____

_____

15 Examine the results in Table 2. What general observations can you make about the distribution of OCP use in cases and controls?

_____

_____

_____

16 The overall odds ratio for the association between fatal venous thromboembolism and current OCP use is 1.6. What do you conclude about OCP use as a possible risk factor?

_____

_____

_____

_____

_____

_____

_____

DISCUSSION

Now read the discussion which follows.

Because of the commonly known hypothesis of the study, and the way that the controls were selected, it was not possible to blind interviewers or general practitioners either to the hypothesis or to whether a woman was a case or control. However, the data collected at the interview were taken direct from contemporary medical records, so that bias in recall should have been avoided. Moreover, an almost identical questionnaire was used to obtain information from general practitioner records for cases and controls, so any bias in providing information about dead and living women should have been minimized.

The findings in this study confirm two previously known risk factors for venous thromboembolism; an increase in risk associated with an operation or accident and an increase in risk associated with a history of previous thrombotic disease.

One early case-control study of fatal idiopathic disease found an OR of 8 of fatal pulmonary embolism associated with current use of oral contraceptives,[11] but most case-control studies of venous thromboembolism have concentrated on nonfatal disease and have found OR varying between 2 and 11.[2] One recent case-control study of nonfatal disease,[12] found an OR of 8·1 (95% CI: 3·7–18) associated with current oral contraceptive use, and provided no evidence that the risk was less in women using combined preparations with low doses of oestrogen.

By contrast, two analyses of the Puget Sound cohort study found some evidence of a fall in risk associated with current use from 8·3 (95% CI: 3·0–23) in 1977–1979 to 2·8 (95% CI 0·9–8·2) in 1980–1982.[13,14] A recent analysis of fatal and nonfatal cases of venous thromboembolism in the Oxford/Family Planning Association cohort study found a significant overall OR of 7·2 ($P < 0.001$) associated with current use,[15] but there was a strong suggestion that the risk was less with preparations containing 30 µg oestrogen than with higher oestrogen dose preparations. A gradation in risk of venous thromboembolism associated with oestrogen dose was found in a recent retrospective cohort study. The risk in users of preparations with higher doses of oestrogen and progestogen was compared with that in users of preparations with the lowest doses of oestrogen and progestogen. There was a significantly greater risk of venous thromboembolism amongst women using preparations containing 50 µg of oestrogen (OR = 1·5, 95% CI: 1·0–2·1, $P = 0.04$), and women using preparations containing more than 50 µg of oestrogen (OR = 1·7, 95% CI: 0·9–3·0, $P = 0.06$) than amongst women using preparations containing 30 µg of oestrogen.[16] No such dose-related gradation of risk with progestogen was observed.[17]

Because of the small number of cases, the power of the present study is such that the minimum significant increased OR associated with current use of oral contraceptives that could have been detected with 90% certainty was 3·0. Whilst previous epidemiological studies have shown a strong relationship between current use of oral contraceptives and venous thromboembolism, the estimated OR of venous thromboembolism associated with current use in this study was considerably less than 3·0, and did not reach statistical significance. These data are certainly compatible with the hypothesis that the OR of fatal venous thromboembolism associated with current use of oral contraceptives is now lower than it was in the past. This apparent reduction in risk may be partly, or even wholly, due to the observed trend towards oral contraceptive preparations with lower dosages of both oestrogen and progestogen.[5]

The present study has concerned exclusively fatal disease, and has therefore involved only a small minority of all occurrences of venous thromboembolism in young women. The high level of morbidity amongst the cases in this study (all relatively young women) also indicates that these women form an unusual group. We do not believe that any inference should be drawn from these data about the risks of nonfatal venous thromboembolism.

ACKNOWLEDGEMENTS

The study was supported by the British Heart Foundation, the Committee on Safety of Medicines and Family Health International. We thank Mr Mike Hawkins and Professor Martin Gardner for statistical advice. We are grateful to Mrs Pamela Baker and Mrs Joan White for their work on the administration of the study. We are also grateful to the coroners, medical records officers, family practitioner committee personnel, the general practitioners who agreed to be interviewed, and the many men and women who returned postal questionnaires.

17   Do you agree with the conclusions the authors have drawn from the data they have gathered?

_____

_____

18   Why do the authors caution against drawing inferences about risk factors for non-fatal venous thromboembolism?

_____

_____

_____

Does the paper help you with your problem?

19   What factors would you want to consider in applying the results of the paper to your own situation?

_____

_____

_____

Box 4.2: Confounding

A study may show that alcohol consumption is associated with an increased risk of chronic bronchitis, and it might be tempting to conclude from this that alcohol therefore *causes* chronic bronchitis. However, we would first have to consider the possibility of confounding: that is, that the observed relationship only exists because alcohol consumption is associated with some other risk factor for the disease (such as smoking), not because alcohol is the cause in itself.

We can express this formally by saying that a confounder is a factor associated with both exposure and outcome, but is not on the causal pathway between exposure and outcome. The possibility of confounding is always present in observational studies. Put another way, there is always the possibility that the groups we wish to compare differ in other ways than just exposure status (in a cohort study) or outcome status (in a case-control study). We may know some of the other ways in which they differ but we may not know all of them.

Given the possibility of confounding, what can be done to try to avoid it? The strategies available can be divided into those used in the design of the study, and those used in the analysis of the results.

Controlling confounding through study design

- Restriction: the simplest way to eliminate the effects of a known confounding variable is to not allow it to vary in the study. For example, if we are concerned that a study of the effects of smoking on lung cancer could be confounded by occupational exposure to smoke, we could restrict the study to non-industrial workers.

- Matching: this is a technique very commonly used in case-control studies, such as the one in Exercise 4. By matching each case to one (or sometimes more) controls, using known potential confounders to match on, the effects of these confounders can be minimized. For example, if we know that both exposure and outcome are associated with age, then by matching cases and controls for age we can compare their odds of exposure without the comparison being affected by age.

- Randomization: the only way to deal with unknown confounders is through randomization, but such a process is only feasible or ethical in certain circumstances. Randomization is discussed in Box 6.2.

Controlling confounding through data analysis

If potential confounders have been measured for each subject in the study, their effects on the association between exposure and outcome can be examined at the analysis stage.

- Stratification: this is, in effect, the analytical equivalent of restriction. Instead of being analysed *en masse*, the study subjects are divided up, or stratified, into groups according to the value of one or more confounders, and the measure of association is recalculated for each group separately.

- Multivariate analysis: the most powerful way to deal with measured confounders is to include them in a mathematical 'model' of the relationship between the exposure and the outcome. A number of potential confounders can all be included together, and the independent effect of each can be described using the technique of multiple regression.

Understanding the difference between bias and confounding can be difficult. Brennan and Croft (1994) have provided one of the best short explanations: 'Bias is an issue of study design whereas confounding is an issue of alternative explanations of the study result'.

Where to find out more

Brennan P and Croft P. Interpreting the results of observational research: chance is not such a fine thing. *Br Med J* 1994; **309**: 727–730

Datta M. You cannot exclude the explanation you have not considered. *Lancet* 1993; **342**: 345–347

Box 4.3: Bias in case-control studies

A bias is any trend in the collection, analysis, interpretation, publication or review of data that can lead to conclusions that are *systematically* different from the true state of affairs.

Bias is a kind of error, but whereas the effects of errors which are randomly distributed can be overcome by increasing the size of a study, the effects of bias, which is systematic rather than random, can only be overcome by careful attention to the details of study design and implementation. Bias may affect any type of study, including randomized trials, but case-control studies are generally regarded as being particularly susceptible to the effects of bias.

A discussion of all possible sources of bias would require a book in itself, but some of the most important biases to consider include the following:

Selection bias (see also Box 3.3)

Cases: Selection bias will occur when the selection of cases or controls for a study is systematically distorted in some way. For example, people with the disease of interest who have been admitted to hospital will be different from those who have not been admitted. Conclusions based on the former group may not apply to the latter. Indeed, if the hospital admission of cases is influenced by knowledge of exposure to a possible risk factor, then our estimate of the association between that risk factor and case status will be biased.

Controls: Ideally, controls should be selected from the 'same population' as the cases. However, it may not be obvious what the 'same population' would be. For instance, it is very common for cases to be identified from hospital admissions. Should the control group then consist of other hospital patients without the condition of interest, or of people who live nearby the cases but who have not been admitted to hospital? These two choices of control population may turn out to be quite different in their exposure to the possible causes of disease, and would therefore lead to quite different conclusions.

Bias in the measurement of exposure

Measurement bias is common, and may originate from the researchers, the method of data collection, or the subjects of the study.

For example, an investigator who knows the disease status of a subject may be biased in assessing their exposure to possible causes of that disease. In case-control studies, measurement of exposure often depends on individuals remembering past events. Patients with the disease of interest may be more inclined to remember or report possible exposures than those without the disease. This is termed 'recall bias'.

Measurement bias is best overcome by blinding – that is, by ensuring that the person recording information about the exposure status of a subject is unaware of their outcome status (or *vice versa*). If this is not possible, standardized data collection procedures should be used for all subjects.

Where to find out more

Sackett DL. Bias in analytic research. *J Chron Dis* 1979; **32**: 51–63
Sitthi-amorn C and Poshyachinda V. Bias. *Lancet* 1993; **342**: 286–288

20   Has the paper helped to solve the problem you started with?

The abstract of the paper is given below.

Abstract

A case-control study of fatal venous thromboembolism in young women is described. Sixty women aged between 16 and 39 who died from thromboembolism in England and Wales between 1986 and 1988 were included in the study. Two living controls matched for age and martial status were sought from the records of the general practitioner with whom each case was registered. Some 115 controls were included in the study. The cases had a significantly higher prevalence of a history of major illness, particularly thrombotic episodes, than the controls. The odds ratio (OR) of a fatal thromboembolism in women who had a history of venous thrombosis was 4·0 (95% CI: 1·4–11·5). There was also a significantly higher frequency of a recent operation or accident amongst the cases than the controls (OR = 11·1, 95% CI: 1·3–92·5). There was no significant excess of oral contraceptive use amongst the cases. The overall OR associated with current use of oral contraceptives was 1·6 (95% CI: 0·7–3·4), while the corresponding OR for 'idiopathic' disease was 2·1 (95% CI: 0·8–5·2). These risks are considerably smaller than those observed in previous studies. The observed risk may be low because the dosage of oestrogen in modern oral contraceptive preparations has been reduced, but it may also be because the cases of fatal venous thromboembolism included in this study represent only a small proportion of all cases of venous thromboembolism; a disease which is rarely fatal in young women. These results cannot necessarily be extrapolated to nonfatal venous thromboembolism.

21   Is the abstract an adequate summary of the findings of the paper?

Title

Risk Factors for Fatal Venous Thromboembolism in Young Women: A Case-Control Study   Margaret Thorogood,* Jim Mann,†
Michael Murphy* and Martin Vessey* (*Revised version received July 1991*) International Journal of Epidemiology 1992; **21:** 48–52.
* Department of Public Health and Primary Care, University of Oxford, Gibson Building, Radcliffe Infirmary, Oxford OX2 6HE, UK.
† Department of Human Nutrition, University of Otago, PO Box 56, Dunedin, New Zealand.

References

1. Royal College of General Practitioners'. Oral contraception and thromboembolic disease. *J Roy Coll Gen Pract* 1967; **13:** 267–79

2. Vessey MP. Female hormones and vascular disease—an epidemiological overview. *Br J Family Planning* 1980; **6:** (Suppl): 1–12

3. Notelovitz M, Kitchens CS, Coone L, McKenzie L, and Carter R. Low-dose oral contraceptive usage and coagulation. *Am J Obstet Gynecol* 1981; **141:** 71–75

4. Kelleher CC. Clinical aspects of the relationship between oral contraceptives and abnormalities of the haeomostatic system: Relation to the development of cardiovascular disease. *Am J Obstet Gynecol* 1990; **163:** 392–95

5. Bonnar J. Coagulation effects of oral contraception. *Am J Obstet and Gyn* 1987; **157:** 1042–48

6. Thorogood M and Vessey MP. Trends in use of oral contraceptives in Britain. *Br J Family Planning* 1990; **16:** 41–53

7. Thorogood M, Mann J, Murphy M, and Vessey M. Is oral contraceptive use still associated with an increased risk of fatal myocardial infarction? Report of a case-control study (In preparation)

8. Breslow NE and Day NE. *Statistical Methods in Cancer Research. Vol. 1. The analysis of case-control studies.* Lyon: International Agency for Research on Cancer 1980

9. Anonymous. *EGRET* Seattle: Statistics and Epidemiology Research Corporation, 1989

10. Anonymous. *POWER* Pasadena: Epicenter Software, 1987

11. Inman WHW and Vessey MP. Investigation of deaths from pulmonary, coronary and cerebral thrombosis and embolism in women of child-bearing age: *Br Med J* 1968; **2:** 193–99

12. Helmrich SP, Rosenberg L, Kaufman DW, Strom B, and Shapiro S. Venous thromboembolism in relation to oral contraceptive use. *Obstet Gynecol* 1987; **69:** 91–95

13. Porter JB, Hunter JR, Danielson DA, Jick H, and Stergachis A. Oral contraceptives and non-fatal vascular disease—Recent experience. *Obstet Gynecol* 1982; **59:** 299–302

14. Porter JB, Hunter JR, Jick H, and Stergachis A. Oral Contraceptives and non-fatal Vascular Disease. *Obstet Gynecol* 1985; **66:** 1–4

15. Vessey MP, Mant D, Smith A, and Yeates D. Oral contraceptives and venous thromboembolism: findings in a large prospective study. *Br Med J* 1986; **292:** 526

16. Gerstman BB, Piper JM, Tomita DK, Ferguson WJ, Stadel BV, and Lundin FE. Oral contraceptive estrogen dose and the risk of deep venous thromboembolic disease. *Am J Epidemiol* 1991; **133:** 32–37

17. Gerstman BB, Piper JM, Freiman JP. *et al.* Oral contraceptive oestrogen and progestin potencies and the incidence of deep venous thromboembolism. *Int J Epidemiol* 1990; **19:** 931–36

Complete the checklist

Now use the answers you have already given to complete the following checklist and assign a score to this paper. There is space for you to add comments about the paper before you decide your final score.

If you wish, you can compare your score and comments with ours, which you will find in the answers section at the back of the book. If you have access to the World Wide Web (via the Internet) you can also compare your scores with those of other readers of this book. Details of how to do this are given in Appendix III.

The checklist is designed to be generalized to other papers of this type. A full set of blank checklists is included at the end of the book, which can be copied for use with other papers.

RATING SCALE 3 FOR ARTICLE ON CAUSATION (OR HARM)

	Yes	Unclear/ possibly	No	Not applicable
		Ring the appropriate code		
RESULTS				
1 Is an estimate of association between exposure and outcome given?	2	1	0	N/A
2 Is it of clinical importance?	2	1	0	N/A
3 Is it sufficiently precise to be useful?	2	1	0	N/A
VALIDITY				
Selection				
4 Was the diagnosis of the disease well defined?	2	1	0	N/A
5 Was the source of the cases/cohort described?	2	1	0	N/A
6 Were efforts made to ensure complete ascertainment of cases?	2	1	0	N/A
Measurement				
7 Were all subjects accounted for?	2	1	0	N/A
8 Were losses to follow-up/refusals low (<10%)?	2	1	0	N/A
9 Were outcomes and/or exposures measured alike in all groups?	2	1	0	N/A
10 Was assessment of exposure objective?	2	1	0	N/A
Statistical analysis				
11 Were additional factors allowed for?	2	1	0	N/A
12 Were appropriate methods used?	2	1	0	N/A
13 Were any 'unusual' methods explained or justified?	2	1	0	N/A
14 Was a 'dose–response' gradient demonstrated?	2	1	0	N/A
15 Was the temporal relationship correct?	2	1	0	N/A
UTILITY				
16 Do the results help me choose treatments or avoid exposures?	2	1	0	N/A
17 Do the results help me reassure/counsel patients?	2	1	0	N/A

TOTAL (add ringed scores above): _____ **(A)**

No. of questions which actually applied to this article (maximum = 17): _____ **(B)**

Maximum possible score (2 × B): _____ **(C)**

OVERALL RATING (A/C expressed as a percentage): _____ %

COMMENTS:

EXERCISE 5   A further paper on causation of disease

LEARNING OBJECTIVES

After working through this exercise, you should be able to:

A   Summarize and critically appraise a paper on causation of a disease.

B   Explain how the results in such a paper might apply to a clinical problem.

C   Perform and interpret simple calculations found in such a paper.

KEY POINTS

- Cohorts may be compared with one another or with the general population.

- Cohorts may differ in more than just their exposure status.

- 'Person-years at risk' quantifies the exposure of a cohort.

- Statistical significance is not the same as clinical importance.

CLINICAL RELEVANCE

- How can I advise patients to stay healthy?

- Does this treatment carry any risks?

THE CLINICAL PROBLEM

You are the senior house officer of a medical team specializing in gastroenterology in a large general hospital. A 55-year-old man with inflammatory bowel disease is about to be started on azathioprine by the Consultant. The Registrar, who has just returned from a conference, recalls a presentation there at which a risk of neoplasia was suggested. Before considering alternatives to azathioprine, which has been used here in this situation for many years, the Consultant asks you to review the literature.

A POSSIBLE SOLUTION

1 Based on the above clinical scenario, write a question, in terms of 'patient', 'intervention' and 'outcome', which could be used as the starting point for a MEDLINE search.

_____

_____

_____

_____

_____

Your search yields only a single paper which you can access within a reasonable time.

INTRODUCTION

Read the introduction to this paper, reproduced below, and then answer the questions which follow.

It is well established that the risk of various malignant disorders is higher in transplant recipients than in the general population. Two prospective studies of transplant recipients on immunosuppressive therapy (mainly azathioprine) reported significant excesses of non-Hodgkin lymphoma (NHL), squamous-cell skin cancer, and primary liver cancer.[1,2] Non-transplant patients who receive immunosuppressive drugs (mainly azathioprine) also show increased frequencies of these malignant disorders.[3] Even though the frequency of NHL is higher in rheumatoid arthritis than in the general population, the rate associated with immunosuppressive treatment is significantly greater.[4]

The risk of neoplasia in patients treated with azathioprine for inflammatory bowel disease has not been studied specifically. The increasing use of azathioprine (or its metabolite 6-mercaptopurine) in this setting makes such a study important. We have investigated the frequency of malignant disorders in a large population of patients with inflammatory bowel disease who received a standard dose of azathioprine at one hospital and were followed up for a median of 9 years (range 2 weeks to 29 years).

2 On the basis of this introduction, what is the research question (patient/intervention/outcome) you expect the paper to answer?

_____

_____

_____

_____

_____

3 How close is the match between the question you want answered and the question addressed in the paper?

_____

_____

_____

PATIENTS AND METHODS

Now read the patients and methods section.

Since the introduction of azathioprine for treatment of inflammatory bowel disease at St Mark's Hospital, London, in 1962, a prospective register has been maintained of all patients who receive the drug and any complications are noted. We abstracted from case records details of the primary disease, including extent and duration of azathioprine treatment. A standard dose of 2 mg/kg daily was used. Details of any malignant disorder and deaths were noted. We sought information about patients who no longer attended the hospital from the referring general practitioner or current consultant physician. If cancer was present, relevant pathology reports were sought. If the required details could not be obtained in this way, the patient's current general practitioner was traced through the local Family Health Service Authority. When we could not find out whether a patient was still alive, he or she was identified in the National Health Service Central Register, which records death and cancer registration. Details of all causes of deaths were sought.

Observed numbers of deaths from all causes and from all neoplastic disorders before the age of 85 and before Dec 31, 1991, were compared with the numbers expected, calculated by applying national mortality rates specific for age, sex, and calendar period to the corresponding person-years at risk up to age 85. Numbers of cancer cases before age 85 were compared with those expected, calculated in the same way as for deaths but with rates recorded by the South Thames Cancer Registry as reference rates. Events after age 84 were excluded from the analysis, as is customary, because of the unreliability of applying reference rates to this open-ended age group.

We also compared rates of colorectal cancer in the subgroup of patients with chronic extensive ulcerative colitis (disease duration longer than 10 years and inflammation extending proximal to the hepatic flexure); 86 azathioprine-treated patients were compared with a similar group who had not received the drug (180). This group was identified from a separate register maintained prospectively at St Mark's Hospital since 1971 of patients with chronic extensive ulcerative colitis undergoing both clinical and endoscopic surveillance. Details of colorectal cancer are routinely recorded in this register. In this analysis of person-years at risk, the date of colectomy formed an additional endpoint. No such prospective register has been maintained for patients with Crohn's disease.

Observed and expected numbers were compared and tested for significance by two-sided t tests, assuming a Poisson distribution; 95% CI were calculated.

4 How did the investigators identify their first cohort of patients with inflammatory bowel disease treated with azathioprine?

_____

5 How were characteristics of the original disease and details of azathioprine treatment obtained?

_____

Box 5.1: Statistical significance

In any study, there is the possibility that any differences we observe between groups (samples) of patients may simply have occurred as the result of chance. The concept of statistical significance helps us to decide, in a particular study, whether it is reasonable to attribute such differences to chance or whether it is more likely that the populations which these represent really do differ.

To do this we begin, rather perversely (but see Altman and Gore, 1982), with a **null hypothesis** which asserts that there is no difference between the populations.

For example, if we wonder whether the prevalence of left-handedness differs between the sexes, our null hypothesis (denoted by H_0) would state:

H_0: Proportion of left-handedness among all males

= Proportion of left-handedness among all females

The purpose of statistical significance testing is to help us decide whether to reject (not believe) the null hypothesis. We make the decision on the basis of quantitative information on the risk of rejecting the null hypothesis when it is actually true (a 'Type 1' statistical error).

Strictly, we should decide in advance the level of risk we are prepared to take that we will make this kind of error (which can never be completely eliminated). Conventionally a 1 in 20 chance or $P = 0.05$ is used.

Then, if a smaller risk ($P = 0.01$, for example) is calculated in the test we may reject the null hypothesis, knowing that if the null hypothesis is actually true, only rarely would we falsely reject it if we regularly use this rule of thumb.

What is a 'P value'?

This is the risk (probability) calculated in a test of statistical significance that, *if the null hypothesis is actually true*, we then (falsely) reject it.

It is not, as is often misquoted, simply the probability of falsely rejecting the null hypothesis, but the probability of doing so if it is true. The difference is subtle but important. In other words, it is the probability, if the null hypothesis is true, of getting at least as extreme a result as that which we have observed.

In particular, a P value of 0.01 (for example) is not, as many examination answers will have it, the probability that the null hypothesis is true; nor does it indicate that we are 99% sure that the null hypothesis is false!

What does statistically significant at the 5% (1% or 0·1%) level mean?

P values are usually considered in broad bands. Four such common bands are given below, along with corresponding levels of statistical significance:

P value range	Example value	Significance level	Sometimes (decreasingly) called	Sometimes shown as
$P > 0.05$	$P = 0.0748$	Not significant at the 5% level	Not statistically significant†	NS
$0.01 < P < 0.05$	$P = 0.0397$	Significant at the 5% level	Statistically significant	*
$0.001 < P < 0.01$	$P = 0.0029$	Significant at the 1% level	Highly statistically significant	**
$P < 0.001$	$P = 0.0007$	Significant at the 0·1% level	Very highly statistically significant	***

† Strictly meaningless without a stated level.

Where to find out more

Altman DG and Gore SM. *Statistics in Practice*. British Medical Association, London, 1982; pp 70–72

Campbell MJ and Machin D. *Medical Statistics: a commonsense approach*, 2nd edn. John Wiley, Chichester; chap 6

6   How were malignant outcomes identified?

_____

_____

_____

7   In this cohort, for what two outcomes were observed and expected numbers compared?

_____

8   In a secondary study, the investigators also identify two cohorts of patients with chronic extensive ulcerative colitis (CEUC). How do these two cohorts differ from one another?

_____

_____

9   What do you think was the purpose of this secondary study?

_____

_____

10   Why do you suppose a similar control group was not used in the primary study?

_____

_____

_____

11   What do the authors mean by the term 'person-years at risk'?

_____

_____

_____

_____

12   Observed and expected numbers of outcomes in each cohort were compared and 'tested for significance'. Briefly explain in plain language the purpose of such testing.

_____

_____

_____

RESULTS

Now read the results section and tables.

Between 1962 and 1991, 755 patients with inflammatory bowel disease received azathioprine; 15 patients received lower doses than the standard 2 mg/kg daily because of myelosuppression. There were 366 female and 389 male patients; 450 had Crohn's disease, 282 ulcerative colitis, and 23 indeterminate colitis. The median duration of therapy was 12·5 months (range 2 days to 15 years). The median duration of follow-up from starting azathioprine was 9·0 years (2 weeks to 29 years), which gave 6975 patient-years of follow-up. 189 patients received azathioprine for less than 3 months because of short-term side-effects, poor response to treatment, or a decision to carry out colectomy.

At the end of the study (Dec 31, 1991) 671 patients were known to be alive in the UK, 11 had emigrated, and 6 were lost to follow-up. The remaining 67 had died before age 85, compared with 58·3 expected; this difference is not significant (observed/expected ratio 1·15 [95% CI 0·89–1·46, p = 0·264). There were 13 deaths from cancer (3 rectum, 3 colon, 1 carcinomatosis, 1 stomach, 1 breast, 3 lung, 1 cervix) compared with 16·4 expected (ratio 0·79, p = 0·459).

Cancer was recorded in 31 azathioprine-treated patients (table 1). This excess over the 24·3 expected was not significant (table 2). There was, however, a significant excess of colorectal tumours (13 vs 2·24, p = 0·00001). 8 of the colorectal tumours were associated with extensive ulcerative colitis, 1 with distal colitis, and 4 with longstanding complicated anorectal Crohn's disease. 2 patients with chronic complicated Crohn's disease developed squamous-cell cancer of the anal canal (expected 0·03, p < 0·001). There were 2 cases of invasive cervical cancer (expected 0·5) and 2 skin cancers. The only case of NHL was in a man aged 89 (outside the age range of the study) who had chronic distal ulcerative colitis and had completed a 24-month course of azathioprine 3 years earlier.

There was a deficit of cancers other than those of the cervix, rectum, and anus (16 vs 22·05 expected) but the difference did not achieve significance.

Table 3 shows the observed and expected numbers of all neoplasms and of colorectal cancers according to the underlying disease and duration of treatment with azathioprine. The excess of malignant disorders is due to an increase in colorectal cancers, irrespective of the duration of azathioprine treatment.

We then compared the frequencies of colorectal cancer among patients who had had extensive ulcerative colitis for longer than 10 years and had or had not received azathioprine. 86 patients who had received azathioprine were matched with 180 patients who had not received the drug by sex, age (within 10 years), and duration of disease (within 1 year). Among azathioprine-treated patients there were 8 cases of colorectal carcinoma (expected 0·26), whereas among 180 non-treated patients there were 15 cases (expected 0·63); this difference is not significant (observed 8, expected from non-azathioprine rates 6·19, p = 0·54).

13   What was the most common specific diagnosis among the patients in the primary study?

_____

Table 1 Clinical details of 31 azathioprine-treated patients who developed malignant disorders

Patient	Sex	Age (yr)	Diagnosis	Extent	Disease duration (yr)	Azathioprine duration (mo)	Follow-up (yr)	Carcinoma
1	M	79	CD	A, R	10	86	8	SCC anal canal
2	F	40	CD	A, R	22	99	16	SCC anal canal
3	F	67	CD	A, R	22	26	9	Adenocarcinoma R*
4	M	47	UC	Extensive	22	2	11	Adenocarcinoma R*
5	M	63	CD	C, A, R	28	31	11	Adenocarcinoma R*
6	M	52	CD	C, A, R	23	64	17	Adenocarcinoma R
7	F	44	CD	C, A, R	16	6	1	Adenocarcinoma R
8	M	62	UC	Extensive	14	84	12	Adenocarcinoma R
9	M	36	UC	Extensive	23	16	8	Adenocarcinoma R
10	M	26	UC	Extensive	13	39	9	Adenocarcinoma C*
11	F	63	UC	Distal	24	6	5	Adenocarcinoma C*
12	M	37	UC	Extensive	17	<1	10	Adenocarcinoma C*
13	M	72	UC	Extensive	52	14	42	Adenocarcinoma C
14	M	63	UC	Extensive	31	12	2	Adenocarcinoma C
15	M	63	UC	Extensive	16	79	8	Adenocarcinoma C
16	F	60	UC	Extensive	26	24	19	Stomach*
17	M	84	UC	Distal	11	5	4	Stomach
18	M	77	CD	Colitis	27	183	16	Carcinomatosis*
19	F	58	CD	Extensive	24	27	14	Bronchus*
20	F	74	CD	C, A	2	1	1	Bronchus*
21	M	60	CD	A, R	23	125	10	Bronchus*
22	F	46	CD	Colitis	19	4	10	Breast*
23	F	48	CD	I, C	21	12	14	Breast
24	F	49	CD	I, C	4	2	1	Cervix*
25	F	35	CD	TI	18	138	12	Cervix
26	F	32	UC	Extensive	13	4	3	AML
27	M	74	UC	Distal	6	5	6	BCC
28	F	39	CD	Colitis	1	<1	17	Dysgerminoma
29	F	60	UC	Extensive	5	10	3	PRV
30	M	54	CD	Colitis	32	20	2	SCC skin
31	M	68	UC	Distal	13	108	10	Secondary adenocarcinoma

CD = Crohn's disease; UC = ulcerative colitis; A = anal; R = rectal; C = colonic; I = ileal; TI = terminal ileum; SCC = squamous-cell carcinoma; AML = acute myeloid leukaemia; BCC = basal-cell carcinoma; PRV = poly-cythaemia rubra vera.
* Died from cancer before age 85.

14   Use the figures given to provide a rough calculation to check the total number of person-years at risk quoted. What assumption is made?

_____

_____

_____

Table 2 Cases of carcinoma in azathioprine-treated patients compared with numbers expected from general population rates

Site	Observed number	Expected number	O/E ratio	p†
Colon	6	1·40	4·29	0·0032
Rectum	7	0·84	8·33	0·0001
Anal canal	2	0·03	66·7	0·0004
Stomach	2	0·98	2·04	0·257
Lung	3	4·01	0·75	0·648
Breast	2	2·92	0·68	0·776
Cervix	2	0·50	4·00	0·090
NHL	0	0·52	—	0·691
Other neoplasms*	7	13·12	0·53	0·097
All neoplasms	31	24·3	1·27	0·186

* 1 case each of: dysgerminoma ovary, basal-cell carcinoma, squamous-cell cancer of skin, carcinomatosis (primary tumour unknown), secondary adenocarcinoma of lymph node (primary tumour unknown), acute myeloid leukaemia, polycythaemia rubra vera.
† Two-sided p value.

Table 3 Cases of all types of cancer and colorectal cancer by underlying disease and duration of treatment

Treatment period (yr)	Observed/expected cases (O/E ratio)		
	Crohn's disease	Ulcerative colitis	All patients
All neoplasms			
<1	6/6·71 (0·89)	8/6·59 (1·21)	14/13·30 (1·05)
1–2	4/3·24 (1·23)	3/1·51 (1·99)	7/4·75 (1·47)
2–5	0/1·91	1/0·99 (1·01)	1/2·90 (0·34)
>5	6/2·74 (2·19)*	3/0·63 (4·76)†	9/3·37 (2·67)‡
Total	16/14·6 (1·10)	15/9·72 (1·54)	31/24·32 (1·27)
Colorectal cancers			
<1	1/0·64 (1·56)	4/0·66 (6·06)	5/1·30 (3·85)
1–2	2/0·29 (6·90)	2/0·13 (15·4)	4/0·42 (9·52)
2–5	0/0·18	1/0·08 (12·5)	1/0·26 (3·85)
>5	3/0·25 (12·0)	2/0·04 (50·0)	5/0·29 (17·2)
Total	6/1·36 (4·41)	9/0·91 (9·89)	15/2·27 (6·61)

* p = 0·06; † p = 0·026; ‡ p = 0·008.

15 For what proportion of patients was information about the final outcome not available? Do you think this is acceptable or a potentially serious source of inaccuracy?

Box 5.2: Clinical importance

Clinical importance is usually defined with respect to the average effect for an individual patient. For example, a 20 mm Hg fall in blood pressure is clinically important but a 2 mm Hg fall is not. At the level of the population, clinical importance has to be given from a public health perspective. For example, if one large population has a malaria prevalence of 25% and another large one has a prevalence of 22%, it may be judged that the difference, though real, does not merit intervention to reduce the higher rate, because of other pressing health problems faced by the populations.

Can a statistically significant difference be clinically unimportant?

With a sufficiently large sample size a real, but very small, difference between two populations can be detected. For example, suppose that we want to discover whether a new drug for treating blood pressure is better than the standard treatment. We do a trial on a large number of patients and find, using a two-sample t test, a 'statistically significant difference' between the mean diastolic blood pressures of those treated with the old and new drugs.

This means that it is reasonable to believe that the difference is real – i.e. that we cannot attribute it simply to chance (see Box 5.1). But it may be that the size of the average difference is only 2 mmHg. This would be insufficient for us to recommend the new drug over the old. While the difference is *statistically significant* it is not *clinically important*. You are most likely to encounter such a situation when sample sizes are very large.

Can a clinically important difference fail to be statistically significant?

Suppose we take a random sample of only five patients from each of two populations which really do have large differences in mean diastolic blood pressure. We may or may not find a difference in mean blood pressure between our samples. Even if we do, a statistical test would confirm that such a difference could quite plausibly have occurred simply by chance – in other words, that the difference is 'not statistically significant'.

In this example, we have failed to show a clinically important difference to be statistically significant. This is sometimes referred to as a 'Type 2' statistical error: the probability, when a difference of a specified size really exists between two populations, of failing to reject the null hypothesis when a test of statistical significance is applied to data from samples of specified sizes drawn from those populations. You are most likely to encounter such a situation when sample sizes are too small.

Where to find out more

Altman DG. *Practical Statistics for Medical Research*. Chapman and Hall, London, 1991; pp 170, 297, 455–456, 457, 461, 464

Box 5.3: Person-years at risk

What is meant by saying that a particular contraceptive pill was observed for 1500 person-years? The total experience of the women using the pill might be made up as follows:

Group	Number of women in group	Duration of pill use by women in this group (years)	Person-years of use
A	100	1	100
B	250	2	500
C	200	3	600
D	50	4	200
E	20	5	100
Total number of years of exposure to risk			1500

In each group, the person-years of use are calculated by multiplying the number of women by the average duration of pill use. These are then added for all groups to give a measure of total exposure to the pill.

One snag is that, in the table above, 1500 person-years of risk could also have arisen from 1500 persons followed for 1 year or 300 persons followed for 5 years. In treating all durations of use as identical, we are making the implicit assumption that any risk of an adverse event, such as contraceptive failure, remains constant over time. If such an assumption is unrealistic, then it is hard to interpret results based on number of events per person-year at risk.

However, the shorter the period of observation, the more reasonable is the assumption of constancy of risk over that period.

What are couple-years of exposure to risk?

With the example of contraception, the incidence of the outcome to be avoided (pregnancy) is related to the total period of use. Because some contraceptive methods are used by women, while others are used by men, different methods are sometimes compared by counting the number of pregnancies per year of use by the couple involved. With multiple partners, the method becomes problematical!

Where to find out more

Hennekens CH and Buring JE. *Epidemiology in Medicine.* Little, Brown and Co, Boston, 1987; chap 4

16   The authors report that, at the end of the primary study, 67 patients had died, 'compared with 58.3 expected'. What do the authors mean by 'expected', and how is the expected number calculated?

_____

_____

_____

_____

_____

17   The ratio of deaths observed to deaths expected was 1·15, with a '95% CI 0·89–1·46'. What does this mean and what does it, of itself, tell you about statistical significance?

_____

_____

_____

_____

_____

_____

18   Assume that these azathioprine-treated patients with inflammatory bowel disease do, in fact, have the same risk of cancer at any site as the general population. Given this, how frequently would you expect to observe seven or more cases of rectal cancer if this kind of study were repeated many times over under identical circumstances?

_____

_____

_____

_____

_____

19   In the light of your answer to the last question, do you believe it is reasonable to assume that these azathioprine-treated patients with inflammatory bowel disease have a similar risk of rectal cancer to the general population?

———————————————————————————

———————————————————————————

20   Which three sites of cancer are most 'statistically significant' in Table 2? What do they have in common?

———————————————————————————

21   What clue does the last answer give to a potential confounding factor in this study?

———————————————————————————

———————————————————————————

———————————————————————————

———————————————————————————

22   Given the results shown in Table 2, does azathioprine increase the risk of rectal cancer?

———————————————————————————

———————————————————————————

23   Now turn to Table 3. For all patients, which period of azathioprine treatment duration is associated with the highest ratio of observed to expected cases of neoplasia?

———————————————————————————

24   Is your last answer modified for patients (a) with Crohn's disease, (b) with ulcerative colitis, or when considering (c) all neoplasms or (d) colorectal cancers?

———————————————————————————

25   Is there a 'dose–response' relationship between azathioprine
      treatment duration and (a) all cancers (b) colorectal cancers?

      _____

      _____

      _____

      _____

      _____

      _____

      _____

      _____

26   How many 'expected' colorectal cancers does Table 3 show
      among how many patients with ulcerative colitis?

      _____

27   We have constructed a further table (see table at top of next
      page), not included in the original study. In this table, first
      check that the data in the second column has been correctly
      abstracted from Table 3. Then, use the last paragraph of the
      results section to help you fill in the missing data (A, B and
      C). Finally, calculate the observed/expected ratios in the last
      column of rows D and E.

      _____

28   Note that in the main study the number in row C of our
      table (expected from non-azathioprine rates) is not available.
      Which expected number (row B or row C) would you regard
      as most suitable to the aims of this paper, and why?

      _____

      _____

Observed and expected cases of colorectal cancer in azathioprine-treated patients with ulcerative colitis

	Main study (Ulcerative colitis, azathioprine treated)	**Secondary study** (Chronic extensive ulcerative colitis)
A. Cases observed	9	A = ? 8 84
B. Cases expected (from general population data)	0·91	B = ? 1· 180
C. Cases expected (from a population of IBD patients **not** treated with azathioprine)	Not available	C = ? 11
D. Observed/expected (A/B)	9·9	D = ? ·26
E. Observed/expected (A/C)	Not available	E = ?
Total number in cohort exposed to azathioprine	282	86

29 Is it reasonable to anticipate that in the main study, the missing observed/expected ratio in row E might, in fact, be closer to 1 than to the value of 9.9 in row D?

DISCUSSION Now read the discussion section, which follows.

An excess of colorectal carcinoma is recognised in long-standing inflammatory bowel disease,[5][10] though not in transplant and non-transplant patients treated with azathioprine. Moreover, we found no significant difference in the frequency of colorectal cancer among patients with extensive ulcerative colitis between those who had and had not received azathioprine. Squamous-cell carcinoma of the anus has been reported previously in patients with chronic complicated anorectal Crohn's disease.[11-13]

Few studies have examined the frequency of malignant disorders in non-transplant patients treated with immunosuppressive drugs. One study of more than 1600 patients[3] found 6 cases of NHL compared with 0·55 expected, and another, of 396 patients treated with mercaptopurine and followed up for a mean of 5·4 years, found 12 cases of cancer, 1 of which was NHL of the brain.[14] The rarity of NHL in the brain in the general population and the very high frequency of the disorder among transplant recipients point to this case's being treatment-related. We know of only two other case-reports of NHL in inflammatory bowel disease treated with immunosuppressive drugs;[15,16] neither was of cerebral lymphoma.

We found no excess of NHL, though our study's power to detect an increased risk of this disorder is small (expected 0·5). It may also be relevant that among transplant recipients, who show the most striking excesses, the need for immunosuppressive therapy for graft survival means that the follow-up period usually approximates to the treatment period. If the increased risk of NHL were mainly related to current treatment (a possibility consistent with the unusually short latent interval), the power of our study to detect an increase would be even smaller, the corresponding expected value being only 0·1.

The slight excess of invasive cervical cancer is interesting since a significant increase in frequency has been reported in transplant recipients.[17,18] Both patients in our study developed the cervical cancer while receiving azathioprine. The overall deficiency of malignant disorders outside the large bowel is not statistically significant and may reflect underascertainment, chance, or both.

The potential risk of malignant disorders from azathioprine should be weighed against its proven efficacy and the effectiveness and side-effects of other medical therapy for inflammatory bowel disease. In ulcerative colitis, when other treatment has failed, azathioprine may defer or avoid the need for surgery. Colectomy, of course, is curative and eliminates the risk of carcinoma in patients with extensive disease. For patients with Crohn's disease who do not need or will not accept surgical treatment, other options are long-term corticosteroid therapy, which is associated with significant long-term morbidity, or other drugs that may be less effective, such as mesalazine or metronidazole.

WRC is supported by grants from the Wellcome Foundation and the British Council.

30 **Look back to your answer to question 2. On the basis of the data collected in these two studies, what light does the discussion shed specifically on the underlying research question the authors posed?**

_____

_____

_____

_____

SUMMARY

Now read the summary.

The incidence of various cancers, especially non-Hodgkin lymphoma (NHL), is higher among patients who receive azathioprine for immunosuppression after organ transplants than in the general population. We have studied the risk of neoplasia after azathioprine in 755 patients treated for inflammatory bowel disease.

The patients received 2 mg/kg daily for a median of 12·5 months (range 2 days to 15 years) between 1962 and 1991; median follow-up was 9 years (range 2 weeks to 29 years). Overall there was no significant excess of cancer: 31 azathioprine-treated patients developed cancer before age 85 compared with 24·3 expected from rates in the general population (observed/expected ratio 1·27, $p = 0.186$). There was a difference in the frequency of colorectal (13) and anal (2) carcinomas (expected 2·27; ratio 6·7, $p = 0.00001$); these tumours are recognised complications of chronic inflammatory bowel disease. There were 2 cases of invasive cervical cancer (expected 0·5), but no case of NHL. Among patients with extensive chronic ulcerative colitis there was no difference in cancer frequency between 86 who had received azathioprine and 180 matched patients who had never received it.

Thus, azathioprine treatment does not substantially increase the risk of cancer in inflammatory bowel disease.

31 **The authors state that 15 bowel-related cancers were observed, while 2.27 would have been expected. How frequently would such a large (or larger) difference between observed and expected values occur by chance alone?**

_____

_____

32 Does the main study alone allow any conclusion to be drawn as to whether the root cause of the excess is inflammatory bowel disease, azathioprine or both?

_____

_____

_____

_____

33 Is the final statement of the summary well supported by the evidence or would you wish to rephrase it?

_____

_____

_____

_____

34 Returning to question 1, has the paper satisfactorily answered the question you originally posed?

_____

_____

_____

_____

Title

Long-term neoplasia risk after azathioprine treatment in inflammatory bowel disease. William R Connell, Michael A Kamm, Mark Dickson, Angela M Balkwill, Jean K Ritchie, John E Lennard-Jones

Lancet 1994; **343:** 1249–52

St Mark's Hospital, City Road, London EC1V 2PS   (W R Connell FRACP, M A Kamm FRACP, J K Ritchie MRCP, Prof J E Lennard-Jones FRCP); and

Cancer Research Campaign Epidemiology Group, Department of Public Health, University of Oxford, Radcliffe Infirmary, Oxford, UK   (M Dickson BSc, A M Balkwill MSc)

Correspondence to: Dr Michael A Kamm

References

1. Hoover R and Fraumeni JF. Risk of cancer in renal-transplant recipients. *Lancet* 1973; **ii:** 55–57

2. Kinlen LJ, Sheil AGR, Peto J, and Doll R. Collaborative United Kingdom-Australasian study of cancer in patients treated with immunosuppressive drugs. *BMJ* 1979; **ii:** 1451–66

3. Kinlen LJ. Incidence of cancer in rheumatoid arthritis and other disorders after immunosuppressive treatment. *Am J Med* 1985; **78:** 44–49

4. Kinlen LJ. Malignancy in autoimmune diseases. *Autoimmunity* 1992; **5:** 363–71

5. Gyde SN, Prior P, Allan RN, et al. Colorectal cancer in ulcerative colitis: a cohort study of primary referrals from three centres. *Gut* 1988; **29:** 206–17

6. Ekbom A, Helmick C, Zack M, and Adami HO. Increased risk of large bowel cancer in Crohn's disease with colonic involvement. *Lancet* 1990; **336:** 357–59

7. Greenstein AJ, Sachar DB, Smith H, Janowitz HD, and Aufses AH. A comparison of cancer risk in Crohn's disease and ulcerative colitis. *Cancer* 1981; **48:** 2742–45

8. Weedon DD, Shorter RG, Ilstrup DM, Huizenga KA, and Taylor WF. Crohn's disease and cancer. *N Engl J Med* 1973; **289:** 1099–103

9. Korelitz BI. Carcinoma of the intestinal tract in Crohn's disease: results of a survey conducted by the National Foundation for Ileitis and Colitis. *Am J Gastroenterol* 1993; **78:** 44–46

10. Gyde SN, Prior P, Macartney JC, Thompson H, Waterhouse JAH, and Allan RN. Malignancy in Crohn's disease. *Gut* 1980; **21:** 1024–29

11. Somerville KW, Langman MJS, Da Cruz DJ, Balfour TW, and Sully L. Malignant transformation of anal skin tags in Crohn's disease. *Gut* 1984; **25:** 1124–25

12. Slater G, Greenstein A, and Aufses AH. Carcinoma in patients with Crohn's disease. *Ann Surg* 1984; **199:** 348–50

13. Church JM, Weakley FL, Fazio VW, Sebek BA, Achkar E, and Carwell M. The relationship between fistulas in Crohn's disease and associated carcinoma. *Dis Colon Rectum* 1985; **26:** 361–66

14. Present DH, Meltzer SJ, Krumholz MP, Wolke A, and Korelitz BI. 6-mercaptopurine in the management of inflammatory bowel disease: short- and long-term toxicity. *Ann Intern Med* 1989; **111:** 641–49

15. Gelb A, and Zalusky R. Lymphoma in Crohn's disease occurring in a patient on 6-MP. *Am J Gastroenterol* 1983; **78:** 316

16. Glick SN, Teplic SK, Goodman LR, Clearfield HR, and Shanser JD. Development of lymphoma in patients with Crohn's disease. *Radiology* 1984; **153:** 337–39

17. Halpert R, Fruchter RG, Sedlis A, Butt K, Boyce JG, and Sillman FH. Human papillomavirus and lower genital neoplasia in renal transplant patients. *Obstet Gynaecol* 1986; **68:** 251–58

18. Alloub MI, Barr BB, McLaren KM, Smith IW, Bunney MH, and Smart GE. Human papillomavirus infection and cervical intraepithelial neoplasia in women with renal allografts. *BMJ* 1989; **298:** 153–56

Complete the checklist

Now use the answers you have already given to complete the following checklist and assign a score to this paper. There is space for you to add comments about the paper before you decide your final score.

If you wish, you can compare your score and comments with ours, which you will find in the answers section at the back of the book. If you have access to the World Wide Web (via the Internet) you can also compare your scores with those of other readers of this book. Details of how to do this are given in Appendix III.

The checklist is designed to be generalized to other papers of this type. A full set of blank checklists is included at the end of the book, which can be copied for use with other papers.

RATING SCALE 3 FOR ARTICLE ON CAUSATION (OR HARM)

	Yes	Unclear/ possibly	No	Not applicable
		Ring the appropriate code		
RESULTS				
1 Is an estimate of association between exposure and outcome given?	2	1	0	N/A
2 Is it of clinical importance?	2	1	0	N/A
3 Is it sufficiently precise to be useful?	2	1	0	N/A
VALIDITY				
Selection				
4 Was the diagnosis of the disease well defined?	2	1	0	N/A
5 Was the source of the cases/cohort described?	2	1	0	N/A
6 Were efforts made to ensure complete ascertainment of cases?	2	1	0	N/A
Measurement				
7 Were all subjects accounted for?	2	1	0	N/A
8 Were losses to follow-up/refusals low (<10%)?	2	1	0	N/A
9 Were outcomes and/or exposures measured alike in all groups?	2	1	0	N/A
10 Was assessment of exposure objective?	2	1	0	N/A
Statistical analysis				
11 Were additional factors allowed for?	2	1	0	N/A
12 Were appropriate methods used?	2	1	0	N/A
13 Were any 'unusual' methods explained or justified?	2	1	0	N/A
14 Was a 'dose–response' gradient demonstrated?	2	1	0	N/A
15 Was the temporal relationship correct?	2	1	0	N/A
UTILITY				
16 Do the results help me choose treatments or avoid exposures?	2	1	0	N/A
17 Do the results help me reassure/counsel patients?	2	1	0	N/A

TOTAL (add ringed scores above): _____ **(A)**

No. of questions which actually applied to this article (maximum = 17): _____ **(B)**

Maximum possible score (2 × B): _____ **(C)**

OVERALL RATING (A/C expressed as a percentage): _____ %

COMMENTS:

EXERCISE 6 A paper on therapy

LEARNING OBJECTIVES

After working through this exercise, you should be able to:

A Summarize and critically appraise a paper on therapy.

B Explain how the results in such a paper might apply to a clinical problem.

C Perform and interpret simple calculations found in such a paper.

KEY POINTS

- Randomization.
- Blinding.
- Statistical power.
- Intention to treat analysis.
- Confidence intervals.
- Number needed to be treated.

CLINICAL RELEVANCE

- Which is the best treatment?
- Is this new therapy any better than the old one?

THE CLINICAL PROBLEM

You are a consultant obstetrician. Several members of your local Community Health Council (CHC) are lobbying for less medical 'interference' in childbirth. A survey of recent hospital confinements conducted by the CHC showed that many women think episiotomy is carried out indiscriminately.

In discussion with your senior colleagues on why you do episiotomies, you consider the case of a woman in labour with a normal presentation of the fetus at 40 weeks' gestation in her first pregnancy. One colleague who recently returned from a fellowship in the USA commented that episiotomy is usual in North America. A second colleague reports from a European country in which she has worked, where episiotomy is used only when there is a clear fetal indication or an immediately imminent severe perineal tear.

A POSSIBLE SOLUTION   You wonder whether you should change current practice. You would like to search MEDLINE and need to select keywords for searching. To help you formulate the question which selected articles should address, fill in the key features of the clinical problem below.

    a   Patient specification:

_____

_____

    b   Intervention/exposure:

_____

    c   Outcome of interest:

_____

    d   Using the above, what is the question you want answered?

_____

_____

A MEDLINE search, using the keywords you have identified, turns up a paper reporting the results of a randomized controlled trial by the Argentine Episiotomy Trial Collaborative Group.

INTRODUCTION   Read the introduction section of the paper and then answer the questions which follow.

Episiotomy is one of the commonest surgical procedures in western medicine and is done in an estimated 62·5% of all vaginal deliveries in the USA.[1] Nevertheless, its use varies widely, in part reflecting the lack of clear evidence about benefits and hazards. In many countries, including some in Latin America, trainees in obstetrics are taught to do episiotomy routinely in the belief that this reduces severe perineal trauma and consequent pelvic floor weakness. Elsewhere, the operation is used selectively for particular indications in the belief that routine use does more harm than good.

We report the first randomized comparison of routine and selective episiotomy policies large enough to assess the effect of episiotomy on the incidence of severe perineal trauma.

    1   Frame the research question to which the introduction leads you to expect an answer, ensuring that you include words or phrases to indicate patient type, exposure/intervention and outcome.

_____

_____

2   How closely does this research question correspond with the question you posed on the basis of your original clinical scenario?

_____

_____

_____

MATERIALS AND METHODS

Now read the materials and methods section below.

The study was from August 1990 to July 1992 in 8 city public maternity hospitals in Argentina, all providing care for women of low socio-economic status. Before the trial, these hospitals had a policy of routine mediolateral episiotomy. The study was approved by the Joint Voluntary Ethical Committees of the Centro Rosarino de Estudios Perinatales and the participating hospitals; all women who took part were aware of the study and gave consent to participation.

Women were eligible if they were in uncomplicated labour at 37 to 42 weeks, nulliparous or primiparous gestation, with a single fetus in cephalic presentation, and had no history of caesarean delivery or severe perineal tears. Random treatment assignments were derived from a random sample generator programme and was organised in balanced blocks of 100, with stratification by centre and parity (nulliparous and primiparous). Each centre was supplied with a set of sequentially-numbered, sealed, opaque envelopes, divided according to parity, which contained the trial instructions. Trial entry was when a woman was moved to a delivery room; the next serially-numbered envelope was then opened to reveal one of two managements: selective – try to avoid an episiotomy if possible and only do it for fetal indications or if severe perineal trauma was judged to be imminent; and routine – do an episiotomy according to the hospital's policy prior to the trial. The trial was incorporated into the routine practice of the participating hospitals. The deliveries were conducted by the medical staff who would normally have been responsible. Episiotomies were mediolateral and done with scissors, up to a maximum length of 4 cm.

The extent of perineal trauma was assessed by the attending physician at the time of delivery. Healing and morbidity were assessed at the time of discharge from hospital and on the seventh postpartum day by an independent physician who did not know the trial allocation. The primary measure of outcome was severe perineal trauma, defined as the extension through the anal sphincter and/or the anal or rectal mucosa (third-degree and fourth-degree lacerations). Based on a literature review[2] and a survey in some of the participating hospitals, we expected an incidence of severe perineal trauma of 4% following the routine use of episiotomy.

Before the trial, we judged that a 50% increase (to 6%) in severe perineal trauma associated with selective use would be sufficiently important clinically to warrant routine episotomy, and we estimated that a sample size of 2280 women would provide 80% power to show this. All analyses were on an intention to treat basis. The χ^2 and t test were used to compare categorical data and continuous variables respectively. The measure of effect was assessed by relative risks (RR) and 95% confidence interval where appropriate.

3   List all the trial entry criteria used.

_____

_____

_____

_____

_____

_____

4   Would you describe these entry criteria as broad?

_____

5   Summarize the two treatment policies under comparison.

_____

_____

_____

_____

6   Was there a formal process of random allocation to these two treatment policies?

_____

_____

_____

_____

7   In practice, how did medical staff determine which treatment should be given to an individual woman?

_____

8   What is the relevance of the reference to opaque envelopes?

_____

_____

_____

_____

9   What main (primary) outcome measure was used?

_____

_____

10   What was the minimum clinically important difference which
     the trial was intended to be capable of detecting and which
     treatment did the investigators expect to give the higher
     percentage of severe perineal trauma?

_____

_____

_____

_____

11   Suppose the trial had been repeated many times with 2280
     women on each occasion in a situation where the true
     incidence of severe tear increases from 4% with routine
     episiotomy to 6% with selective episiotomy.

a   What is meant here by 'true'?

_____

_____

b   In what percentage of such repetitions of the trial would the
     investigators conclude, correctly, that the treatments differ?

_____

_____

RESULTS   Some of the features of the subjects and deliveries in the trial
                     are given in Table 1.

12   Which of the variables in Table 1 are categorical? How similar
     are the two treatment groups with respect to these?

_____

_____

_____

_____

Table 1 Patient variables

	Selective (n = 1308)	Routine (n = 1298)
Oxytocin at 2nd stage	754/1301 (57·9%)	767/1293 (59·3%)
Operative delivery	24/1302 (1·8%)	32/1297 (2·5%)
Birthweight (g)	3244 (427·3)*	3244 (418·3)*
Birthweight > 3800 g	131/1299 (10·1%)	129/1291 (10·0%)
Cephalic perimeter (cm)	34·3 (17·5)*	34·2 (15·5)*
Previous episiotomy	440/1304 (33·7%)	423/1296 (32·6%)
Previous birthweight (g)	3156 (532·7)*	3107 (575·5)*

* Mean (standard deviation).

13 Which of the variables in Table 1 are continuous? How similar are the two treatment groups with respect to these?

_____

_____

_____

_____

_____

_____

_____

_____

14 Are the variables listed in Table 1 those which might reasonably be assumed to be 'associated' with outcome (severe perineal tear?). Have the authors missed any variables you would wish to include?

_____

_____

Table 2 Primary outcome measure: severe perineal tear

	Selective SPT/total	Routine SPT/total	RR (95% CI)	Attributable risk (95% CI)
Nulliparous	11/777 (1·4%)	14/778 (1·8%)	0·79 (0·36–1·72)	−0·4% (−1·6 to +0·9)
Primiparous	4/531 (0·8%)	5/520 (0·9%)	0·78 (0·21–2·90)	−0·2% (−1·3 to +0·9)
Total	15/1308 (1·2%)	19/1298 (1·5%)	0·78 (0·40–1·54)	−0·3% (−1·2 to +0·6)

RR = relative risk, SPT = severe perineal tear.

Now look at Table 2.

15   Examine the outcomes reported for all the women taken together (in the last two rows).

a   Is the calculation of the relative risk (RR) of 0·78 correct?

_____

_____

_____

_____

_____

b   Is the calculation of the attributable risk (AR) of −0·3% correct?

_____

_____

_____

_____

_____

_____

c   The risk of severe perineal tear (SPT) in both the selective and routine samples has turned out to be much lower than the 4% which the investigators had expected in the routine group. Why do you think that might be?

_____

_____

_____

_____

_____

_____

16 The last two columns of the table show the RRs and ARs, together with their 95% CIs, for selective versus routine policies.

a   If there were no difference between the policies, we would expect the RR to be 1. Which of the estimated RRs is/are compatible with a real RR (in the populations from which the samples are drawn) of 1?

_____

b   If there were no difference between the policies, we would expect the attributable risk to be 0. Which of the estimated attributable risks is/are compatible with a real attributable risk of 0?

_____

c   For all patients taken together, is the attributable risk sufficiently precise to reasonably safely rule out a real attributable risk of +2% which the study was designed to detect?

_____

d   Arguably, the last paragraph of the methods section may be interpreted as specifying 1·5 as the minimum true RR in which the investigators were interested. Has this been confirmed? Has it been ruled out?

_____

_____

The final table of results reported by the researchers is given below.

Table 3 Secondary outcome measures

	Selective n/A (%)	Routine n/A (%)	RR (95% CI)
At delivery			
Vaginal middle and/or upper third tear	38/1271 (2·9)	28/1278 (2·2)	1·38 (0·84–2·21)
Anterior perineal trauma	230/1197 (19·2)	101/139 (8·1)	2·36 (1·89–2·94)
Posterior perineal surgical repair	817/1296 (63·1)	1138/1291 (88·1)	0·72 (0·68–0·75)
Apgar score <7 at first minute	43/1306 (3·3)	39/1293 (3·0)	1·09 (0·71–1·67)
At discharge			
Perineal pain	371/1207 (30·7)	516/1215 (42·5)	0·72 (0·65–0·81)
Haematoma	47/1148 (4·1)	49/1148 (4·3)	0·96 (0·65–1·42)
At seventh day post-partum			
Healing complications	114/555 (20·5)	168/564 (29·8)	0·69 (0·56–0·85)
Local infection	9/555 (1·6)	10/578 (1·8)	0·91 (0·37–2·21)
Dehiscence	25/557 (4·5)	53/561 (9·4)	0·45 (0·30–0·75)

n = number, A = number of patients assessed.

17   For which of the secondary outcome variables, if any, in Table 3 is there a statistically significant difference (at the 5% level) in RR and which of these, if any, indicates an advantage for routine episiotomy?

_____

_____

_____

_____

_____

Box 6.1: Confidence intervals

When we measure attributes of, or differences between, samples of individuals we are usually trying to say something not simply about the sample itself, but about the wider population which the sample 'represents'. Our estimates of population parameters, such as the mean, or of the difference between means of populations, will always be uncertain because we can never measure the *whole* population. **Confidence intervals** allow us to express this uncertainty in numerical terms.

For example, in a study of 100 diabetics and 100 controls the mean blood pressure difference between the two groups was 6 mm Hg. The 95% confidence interval was quoted as 1 to 11 mm Hg. This is the interval within which we believe the *true* mean difference between the two populations lies. By this we mean that if we were to repeat the whole experiment many times over, the true difference between the means of the populations would, in 95% of such replicated experiments, be expected to be included within the (various) 95% confidence intervals calculated.

What else can have a confidence interval?

For any population parameter estimated from a random sample, we will wish to see a confidence interval (usually 95%, but occasionally 99% or 99·9% confidence intervals are used) to summarize the precision with which it has been estimated. Usually such confidence intervals will enable us to anticipate the result of a related test of statistical significance. Significance test results alone do not enable us to visualize confidence intervals however. For this reason journal editors often encourage confidence intervals first and significance tests are then optional. Twenty years ago, no self-respecting journal article would appear without a *P* value!

Where to find out more

Altman DG. *Practical Statistics for Medical Research*. Chapman and Hall, London, 1991 (see index)

Bland M. *An Introduction to Medical Statistics*, 2nd edn. Oxford Medical Publications, Oxford, 1995 (see index)

Campbell MJ and Machin D. *Medical Statistics: a commonsense approach,* 2nd edn. John Wiley, Chichester, 1993; chap 5

---

18 For those variables in Table 3 you have identified as statistically significant at the 5% level, use the space reserved to the right of the table to enter the attributable risk (AR), calculated as in Table 2. (Note that the figure of '139' in the table is presumably a misprint for '1239'.) Comment on the three numerically largest attributable risks.

Box 6.2: Randomization

If the analysis of the results of a controlled trial is to be kept simple and transparent, the two or more treatment groups should be as similar as possible at the beginning of the trial. Randomization aims to ensure that known confounders, perhaps age, sex or severity of disease, as well as unknown confounders, are distributed similarly among the treatment groups.

A simple way to randomize would be to toss a coin, if there are just two treatments under comparison, or throw dice (e.g. for four treatments: 1 = treatment A, 2 = treatment B, 3 = treatment C, 4 = treatment D, ignoring any numbers not needed) or shuffle cards. We could also use tables of random numbers or a random number generator on a computer.

Often the randomization is done before patients are admitted to the trial, identifying patients by the serial number to which the patient will be allocated. A list can then be prepared with serial number and treatment group, from which drugs may be dispensed by a pharmacist or to which a surgeon or radiotherapist may refer.

Blocked randomization

Further control over the even distribution of known confounders, like age and sex, among treatment groups can be exercised by stratified random allocation with randomized blocks of perhaps six. With three treatment groups, for example, this ensures that after every sixth patient admitted to a particular stratum (e.g. young females), exactly one third have been allocated to each treatment.

Where to find out more

Campbell MJ and Machin D. *Medical Statistics: a commonsense approach*, 2nd edn. John Wiley, Chichester, 1993; chap 2

Hennekens CH and Buring JE. *Epidemiology in Medicine*. Little, Brown and Co, Boston, 1987; chap 8

Now read the text of the results section.

2606 patients were recruited to the trial between August 1990 and July 1992; 1555 were nulliparous (778 in the selective group and 777 in the routine group) and 1051 primiparous (520 in the selective and 531 in the routine group). 93·0% of women in the selective group and 92·9% in the routine group were assessed when discharged from hospital, and 42·7% and 43·1% respectively on the seventh day postpartum. The groups were similar at trial entry in respect of known prognostic variables (Table 1); nearly all women (98%) had a spontaneous vaginal delivery. No woman was withdrawn after trial entry.

The rates of episiotomy were 30·1% in the selective group and 82·6% in the routine group: 39·5% and 90·7% respectively among nulliparous women, and 16·3% and 70·5% respectively amongst primiparous women. There was no effect on the risk of severe perineal trauma (Table 2). Overall, the rate was 0·3% lower in the restrictive group (95% confidence interval 1·2%–0·6%). Although the overall rate of severe perineal trauma was higher amongst nulliparous women, the pattern of results was similar in analyses stratified by parity (Table 2). The pattern of perineal trauma did, however, differ between groups. Anterior tears were more common in the selective group whereas posterior trauma was more common in the routine group, 28% fewer women in the selective group were judged to require perineal repair (Table 3). Furthermore, perineal pain, healing complications, and dehiscence were also less common in the selective group.

19 Use the information in the tables and the results section to complete, as far as possible, the flow chart below which summarizes the management, observation and follow-up of patients.

_____

_____

20 Is the analysis on an 'intention to treat' basis? (See Box 9.3.) Explain how you know.

_____

_____

_____

_____

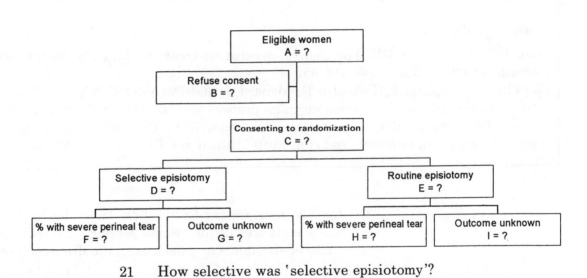

21 How selective was 'selective episiotomy'?

_____

_____

22 Correct the erroneous 95% confidence interval shown in the text by comparing with Table 2, as this is a commonly occurring misprint when ' − ' is inappropriately used as a substitute for 'to' in the presence of '-ve' signs.

_____

Box 6.3: Number needed to be treated

How many patients would have to be treated on the best rather than the worst treatment before one patient would be expected to benefit?

Suppose a new treatment leads to 50% of patients surviving five years after the start of treatment rather than 30% on the traditional treatment. If patients who might have been managed traditionally are instead given the new treatment, an additional 20% of them will be expected to survive five years. If 100 such patients are considered, 20 would be expected to benefit. For at least one to benefit from the new treatment, five would have to receive it. This is referred to as the **number needed to be treated** (NNT).

In another randomized controlled trial, the benefit might be more modest, improving the percentage of patients who can return to work twelve months after fracture of the tibia from 80% to 85%. Switching 100 patients from the worse to the better treatment will result in benefit to five patients. For just one patient to be expected to benefit, at least 20 must be switched to the new treatment. In other words, the NNT is 20.

If the 95% confidence limits are provided or can be calculated for the difference in risk between two treatments then approximate 95% confidence limits for the NNT can also be given: so if the 95% confidence limit for the difference in the proportion surviving five years from commencement is 0·1–0·25, then the equivalent range for the NNT is 4–10.

Where to find out more

Cook RC and Sackett DL. The number needed to treat: a clinically useful measure of treatment effect. *BMJ* 1995; **310**: 452–4

Chatellier G, Zapletal E, Lemaitre D, Menard J, and Degoulet P. The number needed to treat: a clinically useful nomogram in its proper context. *BMJ* 1996; **312**: 426–9

Sackett DL, Haynes RB, Guyatt GH, and Tugwell P. *Clinical Epidemiology: a basic science for clinical medicine,* 2nd edn. Little, Brown and Co, Boston, 1991; pp 205–210

---

23   Review your answer to question 18 in the light of the last three sentences of the results section. Are there any differences of substance or emphasis in the discussion of Table 3?

_____

_____

_____

_____

_____

DISCUSSION

Now read the discussion section.

Before the trial started, we were concerned about our ability to keep the two episiotomy policies distinct, particularly as a large number of doctors were involved. In the event, there was clear separation and a selective policy with a 30% episiotomy rate was compared with a routine policy rate of 83%. This trial is the largest controlled trial of alternative episiotomy policies ever conducted, and provides no evidence that routine use of episiotomy reduces the risk of serious perineal trauma. At the outset, we judged that a routine policy might well be justified if it could prevent one case of severe perineal trauma in every 50 deliveries (an increase of 2%). In fact, the upper end of the 95% confidence interval suggests that, at best it could prevent one case in every 167 women. These results are generally consistent with previously reported trials.[3-6]

The one advantage of routine episiotomy identified in this trial was a reduction in anterior labial tears, consistent with other trials with comparable data.[3,4] In practice, however, anterior perineal tears are rarely a big problem. Any benefit in this respect was more than offset by the disadvantages of a greater need for surgical repair of the perineum, increased perineal pain, and more frequent wound dehiscence (Table 3). We did not set out to address the question of whether routine episiotomy prevents urinary and faecal incontinence. Other trials, however, have failed to detect any such effect. Klein et al[6] did not find any difference between their trial groups in pelvic floor muscle tone measured by electromyographic perineometry, and Sleep and Grant[7] detected no difference in urinary stress incontinence after 3 years.

There is, then, no reliable evidence that routine use of episiotomy has any beneficial effect, and there is clear evidence that it may cause harm. This has obvious implications for the health services. In our country, Argentina, a selective episiotomy policy could avoid about 90 000 surgical perineal repairs each year. On the basis of the current available evidence, a policy of routine episiotomy should be abandoned and rates above the 30% found in the selective group of our study cannot be justified.

Partially supported by the International Development Research Centre, Ottawa, Canada and the Special Programme of Research, Development and Research Training in Human Reproduction, World Health Organization, Geneva, Switzerland. We thank Dr Adrian Grant and Dr Leila Duley from the National Perinatal Epidemiology Unit, Oxford for their collaboration in analysis and manuscript preparation.

24 The authors suggest that a policy of routine episiotomy could, at best, prevent one case of severe perineal trauma in every 167 women. Read Box 6.3 and work through the following questions to understand how they arrive at this statement.

a From Table 2, what is the most reliable estimate of the number needed to be treated (NNT) by selective rather than by routine episiotomy to prevent one case of SPT?

b Bearing in mind the direction of the difference (-0.3%) in the bottom right corner of Table 2, what information can the 95% confidence limits suggest about the most optimistic reasonable estimate for the NNT by selective rather than by routine episiotomy to prevent one case of SPT?

c   Conversely, if you want to continue to believe that routine episiotomy is more effective than selective episiotomy in preventing SPT, what is the most generous reasonable estimate of NNT suggested by Table 2.

_____

_____

25   Do your earlier answers support the conclusion that there is 'no reliable evidence that routine use of episiotomy has any beneficial effect, and there is clear evidence that it may cause harm'?

_____

26   Do you think fetal outcome was adequately assessed?

_____

_____

_____

Does the paper help you with your problem?

27   Returning to the original question you posed on the basis of your own clinical scenario, do you have a satisfactory answer from this published paper? If so, what is it?

_____

SUMMARY   The authors' summary of this paper is given below:

Episiotomy is a widely-done intervention in childbirth, regardless of poor scientific evidence of its benefits. This randomised controlled trial compares selective with routine use of a mediolateral episiotomy for women having first and second deliveries in 8 public maternity units in Argentina.

2606 women participated; 1555 were nulliparous (778 in the selective group and 777 in the routine group) and 1051 primiparous (520 in the selective group and 531 in the routine group). The two interventions compared were selective (limited to specified maternal or fetal indications), and routine episiotomy (following the hospital's previous policy).

Episiotomy was done in 30·1% of deliveries in the selective, and 82·6% in the routine group. The main outcome measure was severe perineal trauma. Severe perineal trauma was uncommon in both groups but was slightly less frequent in the selective group (1·2% vs 1·5%). Anterior perineal trauma was more common in the selective group but posterior perineal surgical repair, perineal pain, healing complications, and dehiscence were all less frequent in the selective group. Routine episiotomy should be abandoned and episiotomy rates above 30% cannot be justified.

Title

Routine vs selective episiotomy: a randomised controlled trial

Argentine Episiotomy Trial Collaborative Group

Lancet 1993; **342:** 1517–18

Correspondence to: Dr José Belizan, Centro Rosarino de Estudios Perinatales, San Luis 2493, 2000 Rosario, Argentina.

Argentine episiotomy trial collaborative group *Steering Committee*   J Belizan, L Campodonico, G Carroli, L Gonzalez, and R Lede. *Hospitals* (local directors) (patients recruited) collaborators:

Buenos Aires, *Hospital Posadas* (M Palermo) (245) C Moreno; J Isetta; N Hernandez; A Cavallini; L Pessacq; M Esteban; D Ortega; P Staropoli; J Dardano; R Tenreyro; L Collada Piris; M Vega; A Candeira; M Rodriguez de la Peña; A Martirena; C Martinez; M Jaureguialzo; C Siamarella; M Damiano; C Godino Conte.

Neuquen *Hospital Bouquet Roldan* (S Cravchik) (147) C Bancora; P M Torres; D Sesma; M C Tovar. *Hospital Castro Rendon* (S Cravchik) (83) V Villaneuva; R Cucui; D Trapote; A Noriega.

Rosario *Hospital Eva Peron* (G Strada Saenz) (70) M Masciotta; A Hallberg. *Hospital Centenario* (C Lavarello) (26). *Maternidad Martin* (J C Nardin) (1153) L Sainz de Vicuña; R Gramajo; E Abalos; D Crosta; J Villa Oliva; A Logica; R Orsi; J Gargano; E Di Orio; R Grado; S Ricci; G Pereyra; P Celoria; M Bagnera; R Waldron; N Bricco; A Golato; N Froyen; R Fontana; H Di Carlo; C Zaffora; R Calcaterra; M Nobile; C Leon. *Hospital Provincial* (H Del Prato) (654) A Tavella; B Ferrari; E Rius; G Abriata; D Baccaro; C Avila; D Nadalutti; R Bugnon; V Aliberti; E Monsalvo; M Frontini; M C Izurieta. *Hospital Roque Saenz Peña* (D De Giovanni) (228) P Premucci; F Candas; M Rappagnini; A Javkin.

References

1. Thacker S and Banta D. Benefits and risks of episiotomy: an interpretive review of the English language literature, 1860–1980. *Obstet Gynecol Surv* 1983; **38:** 322–38

2. Lede R, Moreno M, and Belizan JM. Reflexiones acerca de la indicacion rutinaria de la episiotomia. *Sinopsis Obstetrico Ginecologica* 1991; **38:** 161–66

3. Sleep J, Grant A, Garcia J, Elbourne D, Spencer J, and Chalmers I. West Berkshire perineal management trial. *BMJ* 1984; **289:** 587

4. Flint C and Poulangeris P. The 'Know Your Midwife' report. UK, London: Heinemann, 1987

5. Harrison RF, Brennan M, North PM, Reed JV, and Wickham EA. Is routine episiotomy necessary? *BMJ* 1984; **288:** 1971–75

6. Klein M, Gauthier R, Jorgensen S, et al. Does episiotomy prevent perineal and pelvic floor relaxation? *Online J Curr Clin Trials* 1992; Jul 1; 1992 (Doc N. 10)

7. Sleep J and Grant A. West Berkshire perineal management trial: three year follow-up. *BMJ* 1987; **295:** 749–51

Complete the checklist

Now use the answers you have already given to complete the following checklist and assign a score to this paper. There is space for you to add comments about the paper before you decide your final score.

If you wish, you can compare your score and comments with ours, which you will find in the answers section at the back of the book. If you have access to the World Wide Web (via the Internet) you can also compare your scores with those of other readers of this book. Details of how to do this are given in Appendix III.

The checklist is designed to be generalized to other papers of this type. A full set of blank checklists is included at the end of the book, which can be copied for use with other papers.

RATING SCALE 4 FOR ARTICLE ON THERAPY

	Yes	Unclear/ possibly	No	Not applicable
Ring the appropriate code				

RESULTS

		Yes	Unclear/ possibly	No	Not applicable
1	Is an estimate of the treatment effect given?	2	1	0	N/A
2	Is it of clinical importance?	2	1	0	N/A
3	Is the estimate of treatment effect sufficiently precise?	2	1	0	N/A

VALIDITY

Selection

4	Was the spectrum of patients well defined?	2	1	0	N/A
5	Was the diagnosis of the disease well defined?	2	1	0	N/A
6	If pragmatic, were suitably broad eligibility criteria used?	2	1	0	N/A
7	If explanatory, were eligibility criteria suitably narrow?	2	1	0	N/A

Measurement

8	Was assignment to treatments stated to be random?	2	1	0	N/A
9	If yes, was the method of randomization explained?	2	1	0	N/A
10	Were all patients accounted for after randomization?	2	1	0	N/A
11	Were losses to follow-up low ($<10\%$)?	2	1	0	N/A
12	Were the treatment groups similar in important factors at the start of the trial?	2	1	0	N/A
13	Were all patients otherwise treated alike?	2	1	0	N/A
14	Were patients, health care workers and investigators 'blind' to treatment?	2	1	0	N/A
15	Was assessment of outcome 'blind'?	2	1	0	N/A
16	Was the occurrence of side-effects explicitly looked for?	2	1	0	N/A
17	If yes, were estimates of their frequency/severity given?	2	1	0	N/A

Statistical analysis

18	Was the main analysis on 'intention to treat'?	2	1	0	N/A
19	If no, was a sensitivity analysis performed?	2	1	0	N/A
20	Were additional clinically relevant factors allowed for?	2	1	0	N/A
21	Were appropriate statistical methods used?	2	1	0	N/A
22	Were any 'unusual' methods explained or justified?	2	1	0	N/A
23	If subgroup analyses were done, were they explicitly presented as such?	2	1	0	N/A

UTILITY

24	Do the results help me choose treatments?	2	1	0	N/A

TOTAL (add ringed scores above): _____ **(A)**

No. of questions which actually applied to this article (maximum = 24): _____ **(B)**

Maximum possible score (2 × B): _____ **(C)**

OVERALL RATING (A/C expressed as a percentage): _____ %

COMMENTS:

EXERCISE 7 A paper on prognosis

LEARNING OBJECTIVES

After working through this exercise, you should be able to:

A   Summarize and critically appraise a paper on prognosis.

B   Explain how the results in such a paper might apply to a clinical problem.

C   Interpret the results found in such a paper.

KEY POINTS

- Prognosis: a forecast (prediction) of the outcome of a disease.

- Factors affecting prognosis: the disease, the person and the treatment.

- Beware the 'iceberg' – numbers that do not add up, patients from who knows where?

CLINICAL RELEVANCE

- Doctor, what are my chances?

- What should we allow for when comparing two treatments?

THE CLINICAL PROBLEM

One evening at the beginning of February, a patient's daughter comes to your evening surgery. She is distressed because her 74-year-old father has just been diagnosed as having prostate cancer that has spread to the bones. You have a letter from the surgeon that tells you the man has had an orchiectomy and that at the time of the operation his haemoglobin was 7 mmol/l, his serum alkaline phosphatase (an enzyme found in bone) was four times the normal upper limit and his performance status (a rough measure of how ill you are) is 85%.

The daughter wants to know if her father is likely to be still alive at Christmas. What should you tell her?

A POSSIBLE SOLUTION

The surgeon's letter mentions some research that you might find useful. You visit the library at your local hospital and photocopy the relevant paper. But what do the results mean, and do they help you with your problem?

This exercise is designed to help you answer these questions, and to learn how to apply similar methods to other papers on prognosis.

INTRODUCTION

The introduction to the paper is reproduced below. Read it carefully, and answer the questions which follow.

Since the development of 'androgen deprivation' by Huggins et al., over 45 years ago, hormonal manipulation has been the best available treatment for patients with disseminated prostatic carcinoma.[1] The improvements brought about by new methods of hormonal deprivation are mainly a better subjective response and reduction of side effects, but so far no important prolongation of survival has been observed. The value of chemotherapy remains limited, partly by its poor effectiveness and its side effects.[2,3] New kinds of therapy, therefore, are needed, especially for patients who are refractory to the current ones.

Extended knowledge regarding prognostic factors is essential for the design of future studies. It is important to be able to divide patients into risk groups so that we can select appropriate therapeutic options. On basis of a retrospective study we analyze here the value of various prognostic factors in the selection of treatment for patients with disseminated prostatic cancer.

1   In one sentence, summarize the purpose of the study, in the form of a question.

    _____

    _____

2   List the three key requirements that would enable such a study to be carried out, in terms of the types of subject, the type of measurement performed and the outcome to be predicted.

    _____

    _____

    _____

    _____

3   Why was the study felt to be needed?

    _____

    _____

    _____

    _____

    _____

METHODS

The methods section is provided below.

Between September 1984 and January 1988, 191 patients with newly diagnosed prostate cancer entered two trials organized by the Dutch South Eastern Urologic Oncology group: 75 patients received luteinizing hormone-releasing hormone (LHRH) as a monthly depot (Zoladex, ICI, London), and 116 patients underwent orchiectomy with or without administration of an anti-androgen (Anandron, Roussel, Paris).[4,5] The results of the two trials were similar in hormonal deprivation, and the groups were pooled for analysis of prognostic factors. Of the 191 subjects, 16 with advanced, but local, disease were excluded; 175 patients with bone metastasis (M+, according to the TMN classification) remained.

Pretreatment factors analyzed for prognosis were age, performance status (PS, Karnofsky score), tumor size (T according to the TMN classification, with rectal palpation and transrectal ultrasonography), and grade (according to Mostofi[6]). Laboratory results included were hemoglobin (Hb; in anemia Hb < 8·5 mmol/l), alkaline phosphatase (Alk P), prostatic acid phosphatase (PAP), prostate-specific antigen (PSA), and testosterone. Liver function tests were performed to ensure that elevation of Alk P was due to bone metastases. Prostate-specific antigen was determined with the immune-enzymetric Tandem-e-psa assay (Hybritech, San Diego, CA). Testosterone was measured in 75 patients who were in a pharmacokinetic clinical trial; 59 with M+ were evaluated. Because the patients were treated at different centers, Alk P and PAP were standardized and classified relative to the upper limit of the normal range.

A patient was declared to have progression if his area of bone lesion involvement (entire body) increased more than 25% or the number of bone lesions increased, as compared with the best response.

Statistical Methods

Time to progression and survival, calculated from the start of treatment, were used as end points in this study. Survival was considered with respect only to death related to cancer. To assess the influence of the mentioned above factors, the Kaplan-Meier method was used for estimation, and the log-rank test was applied for statistical testing.

In a multivariate analysis using the proportional hazard model (Cox regression), we analyzed the variables simultaneously with a stepwise procedure (on level $P = 0·10$).[7]

4   Over what period were the patients recruited?

_____

5   Where were the patients obtained from?

_____

_____

6   How many patients were originally available?

_____

7   Why were only 175 patients used for the present study?

_____

_____

_____

_____

8   Complete the following flow chart by inserting the relevant
     numbers, to summarize paragraph 1. For some boxes there is
     insufficient information in the text, so complete these with
     a '?'.

Originally approached for Zoladex trial A = _ _ _	→	In Zoladex trial B = _ _ _	→	Local advanced disease C = _ _ _

                                                              ↘

In this prognostic study G = _ _ _

                                                              ↗

Originally approached for orchiec-tomy trial D = _ _ _	→	In orchiec-tomy trial E = _ _ _	→	Local advanced disease F = _ _ _

9

a   Do you think that these patients were representative of such
     patients in general?

_____

_____

_____

_____

b   Was the point in the course of their disease well defined?

_____

_____

_____

_____

_____

_____

10   This paper was published in 1990. What was the maximum time a patient could possibly have been followed up?

_____

11   Prognostic factors can be classified under the headings of **patient**, **tumour** and **treatment**.

a   Give two examples of each that were used in this paper.

_____

_____

_____

b   Indicate whether these are continuous variables, categories or ordinal.

_____

_____

_____

12   Did the authors omit any potentially important prognostic factors?

_____

_____

_____

Box 7.1: Survival curves

If we gathered a group of 100 patients who had all just been diagnosed with lung cancer, we could plot the proportions alive each week following diagnosis. This plot would be a survival (or survivorship) plot (or curve).

Because the number of patients alive is constant until someone dies, the plot is 'stepped' – each step being the result of one or more deaths.

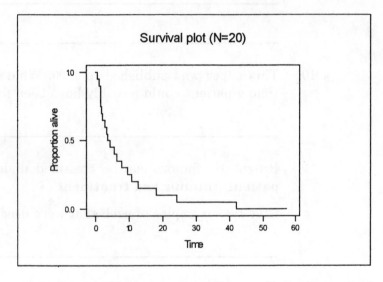

With more patients the plot would become less 'stepped' until we had a smooth curve that approximates the true survival, as shown in the plot below.

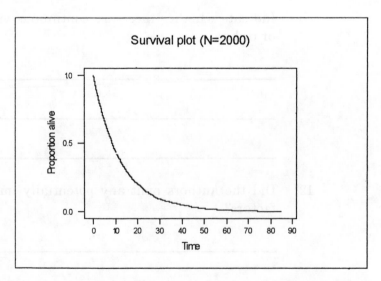

We can use such information to determine the probability of surviving a given number of years after diagnosis.

In practice it is unlikely that a study would recruit 100 patients all at one time. It is more likely that patients will have been recruited over a few years. Because we do not know what will happen to patients still alive at the end of the follow-up period, we say that their survival has been 'censored'.

In Exercise 7 survival is considered only with respect to prostate cancer. If a patient died of some other cause, they would not be counted as a prostate cancer death; yet they obviously could not be counted as still being in the study after they had died. Such patients are 'withdrawals' and are treated in the same way as if we had lost track of them during the follow-up. Both of these kinds of patient are treated as if they too had been censored. We have to make the assumption that the reason for their withdrawal is not correlated with a higher risk of death. Because of censoring and withdrawal a technique called **life table analysis** is used to produce the survival plot.

Where to find out more

Altman DG. *Practical Statistics for Medical Research*. Chapman and Hall, London, 1991
Kahn HA and Sempos CT. *Statistical Methods in Epidemiology*. Oxford University Press, Oxford, 1989

13 Would death from a heart attack have counted as an 'end point'?

14 What outcomes did the authors measure?

15 Were these outcomes objective? Were they likely to be free from bias?

16 How did the authors statistically evaluate the effects of different prognostic factors?

RESULTS   Study Table 1 (see page 118) and answer the questions which
                                   follow:

                               17

                                a   What proportion of patients were lost to follow-up?

                                    _____

                                b   How many patients in the study had died by its end?

                                    _____

                               18

                                a   What proportion of subjects had a haemoglobin of more than
                                    8.5 g/dl?

                                    _____

                                b   Which patients appear worse off, those with a haemoglobin
                                    less than 8.5 g/dl or those aged 60–70 years?

                                    _____

                                    _____

                                c   How do you interpret the *P* value for testosterone (denoted
                                    by 'Test' in Table 1, see page 118).

                                    _____

                                    _____

                                    _____

                                    _____

                                   From Table 2 (see page 119):

                               19   What is your relative risk of dying of prostate cancer if your
                                    haemoglobin is less than 8.5 g/dl, as opposed to more than
                                    this? (you may need to refer to Box 7.3 for help).

                                    _____

                                    _____

                                    _____

                                    _____

Box 7.2: Are two survival curves different?

Suppose you want to compare the survival plots for two groups of patients to see whether they differ. One way would be to compare the proportions alive at a single point in time, for example 5 years after diagnosis. This is simple, but unfortunately only uses a tiny part of the information available. The same applies if you look at median survival (the time by which half the patients have died), but this does have one useful aspect: you can estimate median survival *before* everyone has died, which cannot be done with mean survival times.

A test which uses information from the whole period of follow-up is called the **logrank test**.

To understand the principle of the logrank test, imagine a study in which we are assessing survival in two groups of patients (normal weight or malnourished) in the days following a major operation with high mortality. For each day of follow up we could draw a 2×2 table comparing the survival in each group:

Day 10	Malnourished	Normal
No. who died during day 10 No. alive at end of day 10	a $N - a$	b $M - b$
Total alive at beginning of day 10	N	M

The risk of dying during day 10 in the malnourished group is a/N. Likewise the risk of dying during day 10 in the normal group is b/M.

So the relative risk (RR) of dying if malnutrition is present $= \dfrac{(a/N)}{(b/M)}$

A chi-square test would allow us to decide whether the difference in risk of dying on that day might reasonably be attributed to chance. The logrank test essentially averages these relative risks over all days and carries out a chi-squared test on this average RR. The strength of the association between a prognostic factor (like nutritional status) and death is indicated by the value of the RR: if greater than 1, then the presence of the prognostic factor (like malnourishment) is associated with an increased risk of death; conversely, values less than 1 indicate that the presence of the prognostic factor is favourable.

Where to find out more

Kahn HA and Sempos CT. *Statistical Methods in Epidemiology*. Oxford University Press, Oxford, 1989

---

20   What would the relative risk be if you also had a PS of 50% (compared with someone whose haemoglobin was >8.5 g/dl, and whose PS was 100%)?

Table 1 Univariate Analysis of Prognostic Factors

Factor	No.	2-yr survival (Kaplan-Meier)	P value (log-rank test)
Age			
<60 yr	10	0·34	
60–70 yr	58	0·65	0·44
70–80 yr	80	0·61	
>80 yr	27	0·48	
T			
0	19	0·45	0·70
1	18	0·47	
2	31	0·47	
3	46	0·58	
4	59	0·65	
Grade			
1	21	0·69	0·17
2	74	0·63	
3	74	0·62	
PS			
100%	43	0·72	0·006
80%–90%	73	0·65	
60%–70%	41	0·43	
0%–50%	14	0·51	
Hb			
>8·5 mmol/l	83	0·76	<0·001
<8·5 mmol/l	90	0·48	
Alk P			
Normal	58	0·76	<0·001
−2·5 × U/l	57	0·51	
More	57	0·47	
PAP			
Normal	22	0·74	0·16
−2·5 × U/l	36	0·61	
−10·0 × U/l	45	0·62	
More	71	0·55	
PSA			
<100 µg/l	30	0·79	0·47
100–300 µg/l	31	0·62	
300–800 µg/l	37	0·48	
>800 µg/l	34	0·47	
Test			
<300 ng/dl	17	0·49	0·024
>300 ng/dl	42	0·74	

PS: performance status (Karnofsky score); Hb: hemoglobin; Alk P: alkaline phosphatase; PAP: prostatic acid phosphatase; PSA: prostate-specific antigen.

Table 2 Results of Cox Regression Model

Factor	β	P value
Hb < 8·5 mmol/l	0·50	0·07
Alk P > 1·25 × upper limit	1·14	<0·001
PS		
<100%	0·85	0·018
<60%	0·95	0·022

Hb: hemoglobin; Alk P: alkaline phosphatase; PS: performance status (Karnofsky score).

Our note: *The beta coefficients for the levels of Performance Status (PS) are by comparison with a PS of 100%. The factor listed as '<100%' should be interpreted as PS of 60–90%.*

21 What is the difference between a univariate and a 'multivariate' analysis?

_____

_____

_____

_____

22 Why were they both done?

_____

_____

_____

_____

23

a Which variables were statistically significant on both univariate and 'multivariate' analyses according to the 'conventional' $P<0.05$ rule?

_____

_____

b What P value did the authors adopt for the multivariate analysis, and what effect would this have?

_____

_____

24

a   What do confidence limits indicate?

_____

_____

_____

b   What were they for the relative risk estimates?

_____

_____

_____

Using the Cox regression, the authors defined three prognostic groups, given in Table 3 (see page 122).

25   How could you demonstrate that these groups do, in fact, have different outcomes?

_____

_____

_____

_____

_____

_____

Box 7.3: Allowing for more than one variable

Regression analysis is a way of linking a single dependent (or outcome) variable with one or more measured independent (predictor) variables. If there is more than one predictor variable the technique is described as **multiple regression**. For example, serum cholesterol could be related to body weight and age by a formula of the following form:

serum cholesterol $= \beta_0 + \beta_1 \cdot$ (body weight) $+ \beta_2 \cdot$ (age), where $\cdot$ denotes multiplication.

The terms β_0, β_1 and β_2 are weights (regression coefficients) which multiply the values of their corresponding variable. If the equation is estimated from a set of data, and each coefficient is divided by its standard error, the result can be used to test whether the coefficient in question is significantly different from zero. If it is not, then this amounts to saying that there is no evidence from this data that the corresponding variable, *in the presence of the other putative predictor variable(s)*, provides (extra) information to predict the outcome.

The right-hand side of the equation is called a **linear predictor**. The variables may be categories; thus it is allowable to have $\beta_3 \cdot$ (sex) if sex was coded as $0 =$ male, $1 =$ female or vice versa. The variable coding for sex is called a dummy or indicator variable. The position is a little more elaborate if there are more than two categories (e.g. if race was to be allowed for). In this case separate dummy variables have to be created for one less than the number of categories.

Cox's proportional hazards model (Cox regression)

In 1972 Sir David Cox described a multiple regression type of approach to survival analysis that is essentially equivalent to the logrank test, using a linear predictor based on a set of prognostic variables to estimate the logarithm of the average relative risk over the follow-up period. If there is only one predictor variable, then exponentiating the coefficient, say β_1, i.e. calculating $\exp(\beta_1)$, gives the relative risk for the corresponding variable. If there is more than one variable, exponentiating one coefficient gives the relative risk for that variable, having adjusted for the presence of all the other predictor variables in the equation. Exponentiating the whole linear predictor, for a given combination of values, gives the total relative risk for that combination.

There is no constant β_0 term in 'Cox regression' because this is only required where an absolute measurement is being made. Cox's method predicts the risk only in relative, not absolute, terms.

Where to find out more

Armitage P and Berry G. *Statistical Methods in Medical Research*, 3rd edn. Blackwell Scientific Publications, Oxford, 1994

The authors' method was to display survival plots for the three prognostic groups, shown below, together with the text of the 'results' section of the original paper.

During the period of follow-up (mean, 2·3 years), 92 of 175 patients had progression on hormonal treatment. Of those 92, 82 died, 68 because of prostatic cancer.

The results of univariate analysis of prognostic factors are shown in Table 1. The values of prognostic factors were the same for time to progression during hormonal treatment and for the survival, so only the values for survival are given. Bad PS, anemia, and high Alk P were significantly related to shorter survival. Low testosterone concentration at the start of therapy was also associated

Table 3 Prognostic Groups

Good	Alk $P < 1.25 \times$ upper normal value and PS = 100%
(n = 64)	Alk $P < 1.25 \times$ upper normal value and PS = 60%–90% and no anemia
Moderate	Not in good or bad group
(n = 46)	
Bad	Alk $P > 1.25 \times$ upper normal value and PS < 50%
(n = 57)	Alk $P > 1.25 \times$ upper normal value and PS 60%–90% and anemia

Alk *P*: alkaline phosphatase; PS: performance status (Karnofsky score).

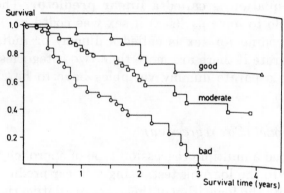
Figure 1 Prognostic groups.

with poor prognosis. Histologic grade was not significantly related to survival. Only PAP showed a numerical trend. As for PSA, no significant relation to prognosis could be detected in these patients with disseminated prostatic carcinoma, although there was a trend to better 2-year survival with lower initial value of the antigen. We could not find a relation of age and T category at the beginning of therapy to survival.

After this univariate analysis, we did a multivariate analysis according to the Cox regression model. All the variables (Table 1) were included in a stepwise analysis. The results are given in Table 2. Performance status, Hb, and Alk P were useful for obtaining prognostic groups. The other variables did not give additional information for these groups. In the case of testosterone levels it could be due to the relatively small number of patients (59) in whom it was measured.

We were able to form three groups for predicting the duration of survival. The good prognostic group existed of 64 patients, the 2-year survival was 75%. The moderate prognostic group (n = 46) had a 2-year survival of 65%, and the bad prognostic group (n = 57) had a 2-year survival of 35% (Table 3 and Fig. 1).

26

a   From Figure 1, about what proportion of men with a 'moderate' prognostic score will live four years before dying of prostate cancer?

b   What key assumption would you have to make in order to estimate the probability of avoiding death from all causes during this time?

_____

_____

_____

_____

_____

_____

c   What is the median survival for men with 'good' scores?

_____

_____

_____

27   Explain in plain English how these prognostic groups are defined and what they imply.

_____

_____

_____

_____

_____

_____

_____

DISCUSSION

At least 25% to 30% of patients with disseminated prostatic cancer do not react to hormonal treatment, and an equal percentage becomes resistant to the treatment within 2 years.[8] New treatments are needed to prevent growth of both hormone-dependent and hormone-independent tumor cells from the beginning and to lengthen time to progression and therefore improve survival.[9] Possibilities of new hormonal and cytotoxic treatment were reviewed earlier in this journal.[10–12] To identify patients with a poor prognosis before the start of treatment, analysis of factors that influence survival are useful.

In our study, PS, Hb, Alk P, and testosterone were found to be of prognostic significance. The importance of PS and Hb has been reported by Berry *et al.*, but they used these factors for hormonally unresponsive prostatic cancer treated with chemotherapy.[13] The unfavorable influence of high Alk P on survival was remarkable and has been established by others.[14–16]

According to Wilson *et al.*, a low testosterone concentration at the start of hormonal treatment is an adverse prognostic sign.[17] Generally PAP is accepted as having prognostic significance, but we could not find a significant influence of PAP on survival in our patients.[18,19] Prostate-specific antigen is widely accepted as the most important factor for detection of prostatic cancer and monitoring of its treatment.[20,21] In our patients with disseminated carcinoma, PSA did not influence survival significantly, although there was a steady decrease in survival with increasing PSA.

Comparable results were obtained by Kuriyama *et al.*[22] Age was not a significant prognostic factor in our study. That result confirmed the findings of Harrison,[23] but Wilson *et al.* detected a worse prognosis for patients younger than 60 and older than 80 years.[24]

On the basis of our multivariate analysis, we defined three risk groups that react differently on hormonal treatment. High-risk patients included those with a disseminated prostatic cancer that is so far advanced that it worsens PS, results in anemia, and raises Alk P. Those patients should be subject to new kinds of treatment; the use of currently accepted standards should be questioned. That is in view of the expected early escape from hormonal therapy, which is more likely to occur with their more aggressive tumors. It is logical to select this group of patients to examine whether early combination of hormone and cytotoxic therapy or radiotherapy is superior to hormonal manipulation alone.

In summary, we conclude that treating patients with disseminated prostatic cancer in a general way does not justify the heterogeneity of response to standard therapy. By statistical analysis, we established the importance of prognostic factors for forming risk groups. Especially for the high-risk group, innovative combination treatment is needed.

28

a   What do the authors feel were the main flaws of their study?

_____

_____

_____

b   What do you feel they were?

_____

_____

_____

_____

_____

_____

_____

_____

_____

29 Use the method of your choice (e.g. underlining or high-lighting) to identify the minimum content of the paper to describe what was done, why they did it, and what was discovered. What proportion of the text have you been able to discard? Compare your result with the authors' abstract given below.

Abstract

A statistical analysis of prognostic factors in 175 patients with hormonally treated disseminated prostatic cancer was done. The prognostic significance of performance status (PS), hemoglobin (Hb), alkaline phosphatase (Alk P), and testosterone was assessed with a univariate analysis. The authors did not find significant prognostic value in age, tumor size or grade, prostatic acid phosphatase, and prostate-specific antigen in these patients. In a multivariate logistic model (Cox regression), PS, Hb, and Alk P were found useful for dividing patients into prognostic groups. The prognosis for high-risk patients on standard hormonal treatment was very poor. The authors concluded that research on prognostic factors is useful and permits a division of patients into risk groups that makes choice of treatment more accurate. The use of new treatment combinations as a start treatment is appropriate for high-risk patients with disseminated prostatic cancer.

30

a Do you think the authors' abstract is a reasonable summary of the paper?

b Are there any claims in the abstract that cannot be confirmed from the paper?

Does the paper help you with your problem?

31 What questions do you think remain unanswered by this paper?

32 On balance, can you use these results to answer the question in the clinical scenario?

Title

Analysis of Prognostic Factors in Disseminated Prostatic Cancer An Update   Peter F. A. Mulders, MD,* Gerhard A. Dijkman, MD,†

Pilar Fernandez del Moral, MD,‡ Ad G. M. Theeuwes, PhD,§ Frans M .J. Debruyne, MD, PhD,‖ and Members of the Dutch Southeastern Urological Cooperative Group

Cancer **65:** 2758–2761, 1990.

From the Department of Urology, University Hospital, Nijmegen, The Netherlands.

* Research Fellow, Department of Urology, University Hospital, Nijmegen, The Netherlands.

† Consultant in Urology, Department of Urology, St. Ignatius Hospital, Breda, The Netherlands.

‡ Clinical Trial Manager, Department of Urology, University Hospital, Nijmegen, The Netherlands.

§ Statistician, Department of Medical Statistics, Nijmegen, The Netherlands.

‖ Professor and Chairman, Department of Urology, University Hospital, Nijmegen, The Netherlands.

Address for reprints: Frans M. J. Debruyne, MD, Department of Urology, University Hospital, Nijmegen, The Netherlands.

Accepted for publication December 19, 1989.

References

1. Huggins C, Stevens RE, and Hodges CV. Studies on prostatic cancer: II. The effects of castration on advanced carcinoma of the prostate gland. _Arch Surg_ 1941; **43:** 209–223

2. Tannock IF. Is there evidence that chemotherapy is of benefit to patients with carcinoma of the prostate? _J Clin Oncol_ 1985; **3:** 1013–1021

3. Seifter EJ, Bunn PA, Cohen MH et al. A trial of combination chemotherapy followed by hormonal therapy for previously untreated metastatic carcinoma of the prostate. _J Clin Oncol_ 1986; **4:** 1365–1373

4. Debruyne FMJ, Denis L, Lunglmayer G et al. Long-term therapy with a depot luteinizing hormone-releasing hormone analogue (Zoladex) in patients with advanced prostatic carcinoma. _J Urol_ 1988; **140:** 775–777

5. Brisset JM, Boccon-Gibod L, Botto H et al. Anandron (RU 23908) associated to surgical castration in previously untreated Stage D prostate cancer: A multicenter comparative study of two doses of drug and of a placebo. In: Prostate Cancer: Part A. Research, Endocrine Treatment and Histopathology. New York: Allan R Liss, 1987; 411–422

6. Mostofi FK. Grading of prostatic carcinoma. _Cancer Chemother Rep_ 1975; **59:** 111–117

7. Cox DR. Regression models and life-tables (with discussion). _J R Stat Soc_ 1972; **34:** 187–220

8. Resnick MI and Grayhack JT. Treatment of Stage IV carcinoma of the prostate. _Urol Clin North Am_ 1978; 141–161

9. Isaacs JT, and Coffey DS. Adaption _versus_ selection as the mechanism responsible for the relapse of prostatic cancer to androgen ablation as studied in the Dunning R-3327-H adenocarcinoma. _Cancer Res_ 1981; **41:** 5070–5075

10. Grayhack JT, Keeler TC, and Kozlowski JM. Carcinoma of the prostate. _Cancer_ 1987; **60:** 589–601

11. Gibbons RP. Prostate cancer: Chemotherapy. _Cancer_ 1987; **60:** 586–588

12. Dennis LC, Hogan TF, and Davis TE. Chemohormonal therapy of metastatic prostate cancer: A pilot study. _Cancer_ 1983; **52:** 410–414

13. Berry WR, Laszlo J, Cox E et al. Prognostic factors in metastatic and hormonally unresponsive carcinoma of the prostate. _Cancer_ 1979; **44:** 763–775

14. O'Donoghue EPN, Constable AR, Sherwood T et al. Bone scanning and plasma phosphatases in carcinoma of the prostate. _Br J Urol_ 1978; **50:** 172–177

15. Merrick MV, Ding CL, Chisholm GD, and Elton RA. Prognostic significance of alkaline and acid phosphatase and skeletal scintigraphy in carcinoma of the prostate. _Br J Urol_ 1985; **57:** 715–720

16. Bishop MC, Hardy JG, Taylor MC et al. Bone imaging and serum phosphatases in prostatic carcinoma. _Br J Urol_ 1985; **57:** 317–324

17. Wilson DW, Harper ME, Jensen HM et al. A prognostic index for the clinical management of patients with advanced prostatic cancer: A British Prostate Study Group investigation. _Prostate_ 1985; **7:** 131–141

18. Ganen EJ. The prognostic significance of an elevated serum acid phosphatase level in advanced prostatic carcinoma. _J Urol_ 1956; **76:** 179–181

19. Babaian RJ and Orlando RP. Elevated prostatic acid phosphatase: A prognostic factor for Stage C adenocarcinoma of the prostate. _J Urol_ 1986; **136:** 1035–1037

20. Wang MC, Papsidero LD, Kuriyama M et al. Prostate antigen: A new potential marker for prostatic cancer. _Prostate_ 1981; **2:** 89–96

21. Guinan P, Bhatti R and Ray P. An evaluation of prostate specific antigen in prostatic cancer. *J Urol* 1987; **137**: 686–689

22. Kuriyama M, Wang MC, Lee C *et al.* Use of prostate-specific antigen in monitoring prostate cancer. *Cancer Res* 1981; **41**: 3874–3876

23. Harrison GSM. The prognosis of prostatic cancer in the younger man. *Br J Urol* 1983; **55**: 315–320

24. Wilson JM, Kemp IW and Stein GJ. Cancer of the prostate: Do younger men have a poorer survival rate? *Br J Urol* 1984; **56**: 391–396

Complete the checklist

Now use the answers you have already given to complete the following checklist and assign a score to this paper. There is space for you to add comments about the paper before you decide your final score.

If you wish, you can compare your score and comments with ours, which you will find in the answers section at the back of the book. If you have access to the World Wide Web (via the Internet) you can also compare your scores with those of other readers of this book. Details of how to do this are given in Appendix III.

The checklist is designed to be generalized to other papers of this type. A full set of blank checklists is included at the end of the book, which can be copied for use with other papers.

RATING SCALE 5 FOR ARTICLE ON PROGNOSIS

	Ring the appropriate code			
	Yes	Unclear/ possibly	No	Not applicable
RESULTS				
1 Is the risk per unit time of the outcome event(s) given?	2	1	0	N/A
2 Is this risk of clinical importance?	2	1	0	N/A
3 Is the estimate of risk sufficiently precise?	2	1	0	N/A
VALIDITY				
Selection				
4 Was the phase of the disease well defined?	2	1	0	N/A
5 Were patients at a uniform point in this phase?	2	1	0	N/A
6 Was the referral pattern described?	2	1	0	N/A
Follow-up				
7 Was follow-up sufficiently complete (under 10% lost to follow-up)?	2	1	0	N/A
8 Were the outcome measurements objective?	2	1	0	N/A
9 Was outcome assessment 'blind'?	2	1	0	N/A
Statistical analysis				
10 Were additional prognostic factors allowed for?	2	1	0	N/A
11 Was validation of the prognostic factor(s) performed?	2	1	0	N/A
12 Were there reasonable numbers of events (10–20 events per prognostic factor)?	2	1	0	N/A
13 Were appropriate methods used?	2	1	0	N/A
14 Were 'unusual' methods justified?	2	1	0	N/A
UTILITY				
15 Do the results help me choose treatments?	2	1	0	N/A
16 Do the results help me reassure/counsel patients?	2	1	0	N/A

TOTAL (add ringed scores above): _____ **(A)**

No. of questions which actually applied to this article (maximum = 16): _____ **(B)**

Maximum possible score (2 × B): _____ **(C)**

OVERALL RATING (A/C expressed as a percentage): _____ %

COMMENTS:

EXERCISE 8 A further paper on prognosis

LEARNING OBJECTIVES

After working through this exercise, you should be able to:

A   Summarize and critically appraise a paper on prognosis.

B   Explain how the results in such a paper might apply to a clinical problem.

C   Interpret the results found in such a paper.

KEY POINTS

- How potential prognostic factors are evaluated and why.
- Magnitude of effect of prognostic factors and the need for validation.

CLINICAL RELEVANCE

- How can we balance the risks and benefits of treatments?

THE CLINICAL PROBLEM

You are a general physician working in a busy medical outpatient clinic. This morning a 56-year-old man has come for a follow-up appointment. He was discharged from hospital 6 weeks previously after an admission for mild heart failure.

He tells you he has remained well since then, and has started back at work, but occasionally notices his heart 'misses a beat'. When you examine him, you find that his pulse is irregular, indicating atrial fibrillation (an irregular rhythm of the atria), but otherwise the examination is normal. Your impression is confirmed by the ECG result.

The patient asks whether his irregular pulse is anything to worry about, and whether he needs any treatment for it. You are aware that atrial fibrillation may occasionally cause a stroke, but you feel that the risk must be very low in your patient, who seems otherwise well. You advise the patient that no treatment is required at present, and discharge him from the clinic.

However, when you come to write the letter to the patient's general practitioner, you wonder whether, in fact, you should have considered prophylactic treatment with the anticoagulant warfarin, in order to reduce the risk of stroke. But warfarin treatment, in turn, carries some small risk of causing a stroke through bleeding.

How can you decide whether, for this patient, the risks of treatment outweigh the risks of inaction?

A POSSIBLE SOLUTION

Over coffee, as you are considering a visit to the postgraduate centre and the library's MEDLINE facility, a helpful colleague offers you a copy of a paper which she feels will save your time. But how can you tell what the results mean, and does the paper help you decide what to do?

INTRODUCTION

Nonrheumatic atrial fibrillation is associated with an increased risk for ischemic stroke (1–4). The rate of ischemic stroke in patients with atrial fibrillation assigned to placebo treatment in recent randomized trials of antithrombotic therapy averaged 5% per year (range, 4·6% to 5·8% per year) (5–7), about six times that of persons without this dysrhythmia (1–4). Within the broad spectrum of patients with atrial fibrillation, the risk for arterial thromboembolism is not uniform, and subgroups at greater and lesser risk clearly exist (4, 8, 9).

Antithrombotic therapy with warfarin (5–7, 10) and with asprin (5) has been shown to substantially reduce the occurrence of ischemic stroke and systemic embolism in patients with atrial fibrillation. In randomized clinical trials, the risk for serious bleeding complications in warfarin-assigned patients has been between 0·8% and 2·5% per year, favoring the use of antithrombotic prophylaxis for many patients with atrial fibrillation (5–7, 10). Patients were carefully selected for inclusion in these trials and followed on strict protocols to minimize bleeding risks. It is uncertain whether such low rates of hemorrhage apply to general clinical practice, particularly during longer periods of treatment and especially in older patients. Characterization of subgroups of patients with atrial fibrillation with substantially higher or lower rates of arterial thromboembolism would help physicians decide which patients could gain greater or lesser benefit from prophylactic antithrombotic therapy. We analyzed clinical features of 568 patients assigned to placebo treatment in the Stroke Prevention in Atrial Fibrillation (SPAF) study to determine clinical predictors of arterial thromboembolism.

1   In one sentence, summarize the purpose of the study.

2   List the three key requirements that would enable such a study to be carried out, in terms of the types of subject, the type of measurement performed and the outcome to be predicted.

3   Why was the study felt to be needed?

_____

_____

_____

METHODS

The SPAF study was a placebo-controlled, randomized clinical trial carried out at 15 clinical centers between 1987 and 1989, in which 1330 patients were assigned to receive warfarin (prothrombin times between 1·3 to 1·8 times control), aspirin (325 mg/d, enteric-coated), or placebo for prevention of ischemic stroke and systemic embolism (primary thromboembolic events). The study design, characteristics of randomized patients, and major outcomes have been previously reported in detail (5, 11). In brief, enlisted patients were those without mitral stenosis, prosthetic valves, thyrotoxicosis, recent (within 3 months) myocardial infarction, recent (within 2 years) clinical brain ischemia, or contraindications to aspirin. Patients were recruited from outpatient and inpatient facilities of public, private, and Veterans Affairs health care facilities and represented a wide array of patients with atrial fibrillation (5). Those medically eligible for and willing to accept anticoagulant therapy were randomly assigned to warfarin, aspirin, or placebo; those who were not were assigned to either aspirin or placebo. After randomization, patients were followed every 3 months to assess compliance and the occurrence of thromboembolism or bleeding complications. No patient was lost to follow-up.

We report on the 568 patients from the SPAF study assigned to receive placebo, who were followed for 731 patient-years during which 46 primary thromboembolic events (42 ischemic strokes and 4 systemic emboli) occurred. Thirteen additional patients had transient cerebral ischemic attacks that are not included in this analysis of major clinical thromboembolism. During the study, 39 (7%) placebo-assigned patients were withdrawn from their assigned therapy and placed on various doses of aspirin or warfarin, in most instances after secondary events occurred (transient ischemic attack, acute myocardial infarction, unstable angina, or venous thrombosis); one thromboembolic event occurred in these patients. The analyses include complete follow-up of all placebo-assigned patients according to intention-to-treat principles.

At the time of entry, a physician-investigator completed a baseline data form, recording associated illnesses, clinical findings, and classification of duration and pattern of atrial fibrillation according to specified criteria (5, 11). A diagnosis of ischemic heart disease required definite previous myocardial infarct, angina pectoris, or coronary angiography (5). A history of hypertension was defined as blood pressure exceeding 160 mm Hg systolic or 90 mm Hg diastolic on repeated observations over 3 months or, if no pretreatment blood pressure values were available, chronic antihypertensive therapy. A diagnosis of recent (within 100 days) definite congestive heart failure required a constellation of orthopnea, dyspnea on exertion or edema responding to diuretic therapy; S3 gallop and pulmonary rales; chest radiographic evidence of cardiomegaly or vascular redistribution; or elevated left ventricle filling pressure or pulmonary wedge pressure at catheterization. Transient congestive heart failure associated with rapid ventricular response to atrial fibrillation was classified as definite if the above criteria were met. Previous arterial thromboembolism included the 9% of patients with either ischemic stroke of any presumed cause, transient ischemic attack, or systemic embolism that occurred more than 2 years before study entry (patients with more recent events were excluded by protocol stipulation). Other specific criteria have been published previously (5, 11). Patients were required to have M-mode and two-dimensional (2-D) echocardiography done within 3 months before entry to exclude patients with mitral stenosis. Ischemic strokes and systemic emboli were identified and reported by physician-investigators at the clinical centers; original medical records that were purged of information about antithrombotic therapy were reviewed by members of an Events Verification Committee, who were unaware of treatment allocation.

Secondary analyses for clinical predictors of thromboembolism involved multiple statistical comparisons that increase the possibility of chance association and negatively influence the validity of the results. Data were analyzed in the following stepwise manner and all comparisons, regardless of the statistical significance, are reported to allow assessment of the potential for finding significant association due to chance. The initial analysis involved eight clinical features prospectively selected on the basis of several considerations, including the biologic plausibility of a relation to stroke risk. The second analysis included five additional clinical features identified in previously reported studies relating atrial fibrillation to thromboembolism (10, 12–17). A multivariate analysis of eight additional clinical features was finally done that included the original eight prospectively selected variables. Univariate analysis preceded multivariate analysis in each step. Echocardiographic predictors of thromboembolism are analyzed in a separate report (18).

Baseline comparisons between groups were performed using the chi-square or Fisher exact test for categorical data and the Student *t*-test for continuous data. Cox proportional hazards regression was used to estimate the univariate risk for a characteristic and for age-adjusted risks. Forward and backward stepwise Cox modeling were done to identify significant predictors of thromboembolism, using the EGRET statistical software (Statistics and Epidemiology Research Corporation, Seattle, Washington). Confidence intervals (CI) for event rates were calculated with Poisson regression analysis (19), also using EGRET software. Confidence intervals for odds ratio were calculated using an exact method (20). All statistical tests were two-sided, and significance was accepted at the 0·05 level.

4   Over what period were the patients recruited?

_____

5   Where were the patients obtained from?

_____

_____

6   How many patients were included in this study?

_____

7   Complete the following flow chart to summarize paragraph 1 (you may have to put a '?' if the data are not available):

Patients approached in SPAF study: A = _ _ _	→	Patients enlisted: B = _ _ _	→	Controls (entered this study): C = _ _ _

8

a   Do you think that these patients were representative of such patients in general?

_____

_____

_____

b   From what point in their illness were patients followed?

_____

9

a   What did the authors mean by the 'intention to treat' analysis used here?

_____

_____

_____

b   Why do you think this was done? (You may wish to refer to Box 9.3 for more information.)

_____

_____

_____

10   What proportion of patients were lost to follow-up?

_____

11   Would someone who had an artificial heart valve have been included?

_____

12   How did the investigators check for the occurrence of an 'event' (ischaemic stroke or systemic embolism)?

_____

_____

_____

13   Were these outcomes objective? Were they likely to be free from bias?

_____

_____

_____

_____

14   For prognostic studies there is a 'rule of thumb' that at least
      10 (preferably 20 or even 25) events are needed for each
      prognostic factor being examined, to prevent the predictions
      from the model being too closely tailored to the original data
      set. How many factors would it have been reasonable to
      investigate in this study?

      _____

      _____

15   How did the authors statistically evaluate the effects of
      different prognostic factors?

      _____

      _____

      _____

RESULTS

Univariate analysis of eight prospectively selected clinical variables showed that a history of hypertension, recent congestive heart failure, and previous thromboembolism were each associated with a significantly increased risk for thromboembolism that persisted after adjustment for age (Table 1). The rate of thromboembolism among patients with any of these features was 9·0% or more per year. Multivariate analyses using all eight variables yielded the same three variables as independent contributors to thromboembolic risk with relative risks between 2·1 and 2·6 (Table 2). Duration of atrial fibrillation, intermittency of atrial fibrillation, and associated ischemic heart disease were not significantly related to the risk for thromboembolism.

A review of the English-language literature yielded five clinical features (Table 3) that were not included in the set of eight prospectively selected variables, but were significantly related to thromboembolism in one or more studies (10, 12–17). Previous myocardial infarction, hypertension (defined in various ways), and age were most consistently associated with thromboembolism in these studies, although the patient groups and frequency of these patient characteristics differed substantially. According to the results of univariate analysis, none of these five additional variables was significantly related to thromboembolic events, although the 95% confidence intervals included relative risks of 2 to 3 for several variables (Table 3). Multivariate analysis of these five variables, combined with the eight prospectively selected, yielded only the original three clinical features predictive of thromboembolism: history of hypertension, recent congestive heart failure, and previous thromboembolism. When the thromboembolic risk associated with eight additional clinical variables was assessed, diabetes, diuretic therapy, and systolic blood pressure exceeding 160 mm Hg were univariately predictive of thromboembolism (Table 3), but they were not significant independent predictors when multivariate analysis considering the eight prospectively selected features was done.

On the basis of the presence or absence of the three independent clinical predictors, risk groups were derived (Table 4). Patients with no clinical risk factors (42% of enrolled patients) had an event rate of only 2·5% per year, significantly less ($P < 0·001$) than those with one (7·2% per year) or more (17·6% per year) risk factors. When patients with minimally disabling strokes ($n = 24$) were excluded, these risk factors were again predictive of thromboembolic events ($P = 0·02$; 1·3% per year in those without risk factors compared with 4·6% per year in those with one or more risk factors). Among low-risk patients with no clinical risk factors ($n = 241$), the occurrence of thromboembolism was related to age ($P < 0·01$) and to diabetes ($P = 0·004$) (Table 5). Nondiabetic patients with no clinical risk factors ($n = 218$, 38% of enrolled patients) had a thromboembolic rate of 1·4% per year (CI, 0·05% to 3·7%). Patients without clinical risk factors who were under 60 years of age ($n = 73$) had no thromboembolic events (Table 5).

Box 8.1: What else to look for in prognostic studies

Prognostic groups

We often want to be able to assign patients to different prognostic groups, such as those with a good prognosis or those with a poor prognosis, on the basis of their clinical or diagnostic features.

One way to form prognostic groups is to convert all variables into categories and then comparing the survival of patients at each combination of levels of the variables. Categories with 'similar' prognoses can be progressively combined, until what is left is a set of three or four well-defined prognostic groups. A difficulty with this approach is in deciding how to categorize continuous variables such as haemoglobin. There is also a risk of losing information by an inappropriate cut-point, although a formal way of doing this is by using CART (Classification And Regression Tree) methods which have only recently become available for survival analysis (see Exercise 3 for an example of this method).

An alternative is to form prognostic groups from the distribution of values of the linear predictor (see Box 7.3). For example, we might define good, intermediate and poor prognostic groups by using the lower and upper thirds of the observed distribution of the linear predictor.

Validation

Once a prognostic index has been constructed for a set of patients, its performance needs to be validated. How well does it really *discriminate* between patients 'who do well' and those who do not? In general a prognostic index will not perform so well on a second or subsequent sets of patients, because it will have been tailored, as it were, to the original 'training set'. The actual performance can be estimated in a number of ways; one is to have a separate 'validation' set of patients – that is, the prognostic index is cross-validated. Another approach is to degrade the performance on the training set to the level one would expect on a separate validation set (useful if patients are scarce) by a process known as 'shrinkage'. This is unlikely to have much effect if the data set has at least 20–30 deaths per regression coefficient in the prognostic index.

Discrimination

One suggestion is to use a measure of concordance between the relative rankings (for each possible pair of subjects) of the prognostic index and survival time. If the prognostic index is a good one, most pairs of subjects will have concordant rankings. This procedure involves considerable computing effort however.

Where to find out more

Fielding LP, Fenoglio-Preiser C, and Freedman LS. The future of prognostic factors in outcome prediction for patients with cancer. *Cancer* 1992; **70:** 2367–2377

Simon R and Altman DG. Statistical aspects of prognostic factor studies in oncology. *Br J Cancer* 1994; **69:** 979–985

16

a   Give two examples of prognostic factors related to each of the
     patient, the *disease* and the *treatment* that were examined in
     this paper.

     _____

     _____

     _____

b   Indicate whether these are continuous variables, categories
     or ordinal.

     _____

     _____

     _____

c   What potential disadvantage is there from categorizing con-
     tinuous (or ordinal) data?

     _____

     _____

     _____

17   Did the authors omit any potentially important prognostic
     factors?

     _____

     _____

     _____

     _____

     _____

18   On the univariate analysis in Table 1, ignoring the age-adjustment, use the event rate to decide which prognostic variable was associated with:

a   The greatest risk of thromboembolism.

b   The least precisely estimated risk of thromboembolism.

19

a   Describe the relationship between age and risk of thrombo-embolism in Table 1.

b   Now examine the results of Cox regression, given in Table 2. What was the effect of the Cox regression on the clinical prognostic variables?

20   Why do you think 'age' in Table 2 is only given one relative risk although in Table 1 there are three (age 60 or under has an implied RR of 1)?

21   The authors defined three prognostic groups (see Table 4, page 140). How would they classify someone:

a   With a history of hypertension and recent congestive heart failure?

Table 1 Univariate Analyses of Prospectively Selected Features and Thromboembolism

Variable*	Number of Patients	Number of Events	Event Rate†	Relative Risk	95% CI	Age-adjusted Relative Risk	95% CI
Age							
≤60 years	127	9	5·7				
61 to 75 years	311	24	5·9	1·0	0·5 to 2·2		
≥76 years	130	13	8·0	1·3	0·6 to 3·1		
History of hypertension	295	34	9·0	2·6	1·4 to 5·0	2·5	1·3 to 4·8
Duration of atrial fibrillation ≥ 1 year	388	30	5·9	0·7	0·4 to 1·4	0·7	0·4 to 1·3
Intermittent atrial fibrillation	196	14	5·6	0·9	0·5 to 1·6	0·9	0·5 to 1·8
Definite history of congestive heart failure	111	14	10·3	1·9	1·0 to 3·6	1·8	1·0 to 3·4
Recent congestive heart failure	57	9	17·7	3·2	1·5 to 6·7	3·1	1·5 to 6·4
Previous thromboembolism	49	10	14·6	2·7	1·3 to 5·4	2·6	1·3 to 5·2
Ischemic heart disease	81	8	6·7	1·1	0·5 to 2·4	1·0	0·5 to 2·2

* *See* Methods section for definition of variables.

† Percent per patient-year of follow-up.

Table 2 Multivariate Analyses of Prospectively Selected Features and Thromboembolism

Variable	Relative Risk	95% CI	P Value
Age*	1·2	0·9 to 1·6	>0·2
History of hypertension	2·2	1·1 to 4·3	0·02
Previous thromboembolism	2·1	1·0 to 4·2	0·04
Recent congestive heart failure	2·6	1·2 to 5·4	0·01

* Risk by decade; age forced into the Cox proportional hazards model.

b Aged 67 with neither of the above?

_____

c How else could they have demonstrated that these groups do have different outcomes?

_____

22   The risk of thromboembolism in people with no risk factors is 2.5% per person per year. The mean number of years per person until such an event is $100/2\cdot5 = 40$ years (compare with NNT in the therapy exercise).

a   Calculate the mean number of years per person and corresponding confidence limits for the other risk groups.

_____

_____

_____

b   Using your answers to the last question, indicate for each risk group whether it would be unusual for someone to develop a thromboembolism within 4 years?

_____

_____

_____

23   When might age be important?

_____

_____

DISCUSSION

Identification of subgroups of patients with atrial fibrillation with higher or lower risk for arterial thromboembolism may importantly influence decisions regarding antithrombotic prophylaxis. This analysis revealed three clinical variables that independently predicted a higher risk for thromboembolism: history of hypertension (relative risk, 2·2), recent congestive heart failure (relative risk, 2·6), and previous thromboembolism (relative risk, 2·1). Over half of the patients in the SPAF study had one or more of these features. The thromboembolic event rate in these patients exceeded 7% per year. Except in low-risk patients, age was not an independent predictor of thromboembolism.

Multiple secondary analyses involving subgroups are notoriously unreliable because the likelihood of finding significant differences in event rates between groups increases with each comparison and because insufficient power often limits the value of statistically insignificant results (21, 22). The validity of the results of secondary analyses depends on the level of statistical significance, the sequence and multiplicity of analyses, and the biologic plausibility of the findings. The stepwise approach to our analyses and the detailed reporting of complete rather than selected results allow evaluation of both alpha and beta errors. Each step is increasingly exploratory for purposes of generating hypotheses, requiring independent verification and mitigated by pathophysiologic concepts. Given the cost, effort, and patient risk involved in obtaining these data, dismissing all results of secondary analyses as inherently invalid seems unwise, but the findings must be interpreted with appropriate caution.

Differences in definition of variables (often not provided), study design, antithrombotic therapy, and specific statistical methods confound direct comparison of predictors of arterial thromboembolism from previously reported studies (10, 12–17). Results are often stated as not significant for a given variable, but the power to exclude a clinically important association may not be provided. Predictors of arterial thromboembolism may vary with patient age, sex, or duration of follow-up, and be influenced by the inclusion

Table 3 Secondary Variables and Thromboembolism

Variable	Number of Patients	Number of Events	Event Rate*	Univariate Relative Risk	95% CI	Age-adjusted Relative Risk	95% CI
Literature-derived variables							
Female sex	170	16	7·5	1·2	0·7 to 2·3	1·2	0·6 to 2·1
Systolic hypertension†	167	18	8·1	1·5	0·8 to 2·7	1·3	0·7 to 2·4
Diastolic hypertension	85	10	9·3	1·6	0·8 to 3·2	1·5	0·7 to 3·0
Previous myocardial infarction	44	6	9·1	1·5	0·6 to 3·6	1·4	0·6 to 3·4
History of definite angina	59	7	7·8	1·3	0·6 to 2·9	1·2	0·5 to 2·7
Additional clinical variables							
Diabetes	105	14	10·9	2·1	1·1 to 3·9	2·1	1·1 to 3·9
Current smoker	90	7	5·7	0·9	0·4 to 2·0	1·0	0·4 to 2·2
Alcohol use ≥ days per week	110	8	5·7	0·9	0·4 to 2·0	0·9	0·4 to 2·0
Diuretic use	213	24	9·0	1·8	1·0 to 3·3	1·7	1·0 to 3·1
Systolic blood pressure > 160 at entry	78	12	12·2	2·2	1·1 to 4·2	2·0	1·0 to 3·9
Pacemaker	31	3	8·7	1·4	0·4 to 4·5	1·2	0·4 to 4·0
Left ventricular hypertrophy by electrocardiogram	55	8	10·3	1·8	0·8 to 3·8	1·7	0·8 to 3·6
Atrial fibrillation onset < 3 months	76	7	8·6	1·3	0·6 to 3·0	1·4	0·6 to 3·2

* Percent per patient-year.

† Systolic hypertension > 150 mm Hg on baseline or 1 month follow-up; diastolic hypertension > 90 mm Hg on baseline or 1 month follow-up.

Table 4 Event Rates by Clinical Risk Factors*

Clinical Risk Group	Number of Patients	Number of Events	Thromboembolism Rate (% per year)	95% CI†
No risk factors	241	8	2·5	1·3 to 5·0
One risk factor	259	24	7·2	4·8 to 10·8
Two or three risk factors	68	14	17·6	10·5 to 29·9

* Risk factors are history of hypertension, recent congestive heart failure, and previous thromboembolism.

† Poisson regression.

Table 5 Predictors of Thromboembolism in Low-risk Patients*

Variable	Patients with Thromboembolism	Patients without Thromboembolism
Number	8	233
Female sex, %	50	27
Current smoker, %	25	16
Age, y		
<60, %	0	31
61 to 75, %	88	46
≥76, %	13	23
Mean age, y	72†	64
Mean systolic blood pressure, *mm Hg*	150‡	129
Mean diastolic blood pressure, *mm Hg*	83§	77
Systolic blood pressure > 160 at entry, %	13	3
Duration of atrial fibrillation ≥ 1 year, %	75	70
Intermittent atrial fibrillation, %	38	37
History of remote congestive heart failure, %	0	9
Diabetes, %	50¶	8
Cervical bruit or carotid endarterectomy, %	13	4
Ischemic heart disease, %	13	9
Previous definite myocardial infarction, %	0	4

* Patients with no clinical risk factors as defined in Table 4.

† $P = 0.01$.

‡ $P = 0.001$.

§ $P = 0.04$.

¶ $P = 0.003$.

of minor events (for example, transient ischemic attacks). Hence, the clinical generalizability of positive correlations and the validity of negative correlations from previous studies remain suspect. Our results do not conflict directly with those of most previous studies (that is, univariate confidence intervals overlap for most variables) (see Table 3). The failure in other studies to include variables found to be independently predictive in our multivariate analysis would probably result in identification of less reliable predictors (for example, age or previous myocardial infarction). The prospective accrual of data before thromboembolic events occur, the relatively large number of thromboembolic events, and multivariate analyses of several key cardiovascular variables in sequence give special weight to our results. The SPAF patient group is representative of the broad spectrum of patients with atrial fibrillation seen by physicians (23, 24). For these reasons, the predictive guidelines derived from this secondary analysis may be the best that are currently available.

Warfarin reduces the risk of ischemic stroke in patients with atrial fibrillation by about two thirds (range, 35% to 86%) (5–7, 10) based on randomized clinical trials with rates of major hemorrhage up to 2·5% per year. Although anticoagulation is effective in reducing stroke, it is not indicated in patients with a low risk for thromboembolism, who may not benefit from such therapy when the risk for bleeding is considered. The low risk for major hemorrhage in patients assigned to anticoagulation therapy in recent clinical trials may not be generalizable to patients outside clinical trials, especially older patients followed for longer periods. Administration of aspirin has relatively lower risk, but its benefit compared with that of warfarin is unclear and is being assessed in the SPAF II study. Patients with none of the three clinical risk factors identified in this analysis had a low risk for thromboembolism (2·5% per year). Such patients comprised 42% of the SPAF study group and probably an even larger proportion of patients with atrial fibrillation encountered in general clinical practice. On the basis of this secondary analysis, large subgroups of patients with atrial fibrillation at low risk for thromboembolism were identified in whom the dangers associated with anticoagulant therapy may outweigh its benefit.

Box 8.2: Poisson regression

The authors in Exercise 8 used this method to estimate absolute risks (strictly, rates) of thromboembolism. If the occurrence of cases of a disease can be described as following a Poisson distribution, then the rate λ at which the disease occurs for a particular combination of age, sex and body weight, for example, is estimated by:

$$\lambda = \frac{\text{Number of occurrences}}{\text{Person-time at risk}} = \frac{r}{N}$$

Poisson regression aims to predict the logarithm of this rate using a linear combination of variables (linear predictor), as follows:

$\ln(\lambda) = \beta_0 + \beta_1 \cdot (\text{age}) + \beta_2 \cdot (\text{sex}) + \beta_3 \cdot (\text{body weight})$, where '$\cdot$' denotes multiplication

The logarithm is used to prevent the estimated rate being negative. Because $(\ln(\lambda) = \ln(r) - \ln(N)$, and r is what is observed, we can modify the above equation to:

$\ln(r) = \ln(N) + \beta_0 + \beta_1 \cdot (\text{age}) + \beta_2 \cdot (\text{sex}) + \beta_3 \cdot (\text{body weight})$

Since r is assumed to be Poisson, this model is referred to as 'Poisson regression'. It is closely related to Cox's proportional hazards model, since as shown by Breslow, the Cox model can be obtained by assuming constant death rates (λ) during each time interval – corresponding to a Poisson risk of occurrence.

Where to find out more

Aitkin M, Anderson D, Francis B, and Hinde J. *Statistical Modelling in GLIM*. Oxford Univesity Press, Oxford, 1989; pp 287–292

24

a   What do the authors feel were the main flaws of their study?

_____

_____

_____

_____

b   What do you feel they were?

_____

_____

_____

_____

_____

25 Create a structured abstract of the paper by underlining or highlighting the essential text in each section, aiming for 200–300 words.

Abstract

■ *Objective:* To identify those patients with nonrheumatic atrial fibrillation who are at high risk and those at low risk for arterial thromboembolism.

■ *Design:* Cohort study of patients assigned to placebo in a randomized clinical trial.

■ *Setting:* Five hundred sixty-eight inpatients and outpatients with nonrheumatic atrial fibrillation assigned to placebo therapy at 15 U.S. medical centers from 1987 to 1989 in the Stroke Prevention in Atrial Fibrillation study. Patients were followed for a mean of 1·3 years.

■ *Measurements:* Clinical variables were assessed at study entry and correlated with subsequent ischemic stroke and systemic embolism by multivariate analysis.

■ *Main Results:* Recent (within 3 months) congestive heart failure, a history of hypertension, and previous arterial thromboembolism were each significantly and independently associated with a substantial risk for thromboembolism ($>7\%$ per year; $P \leqslant 0.05$). The presence of these three independent clinical predictors (recent congestive heart failure, history of hypertension, previous thromboembolism) defined patients with rates of thromboembolism of 2·5% per year (no risk factors), 7·2% per year (one risk factor), and 17·6% per year (two or three risk factors). Nondiabetic patients without these risk factors, comprising 38% of the cohort, had a low risk for thromboembolism (1·4% per year; 95% CI, 0·05% to 3·7%). Patients without clinical risk factors who were under 60 years of age had no thromboembolic events.

■ *Conclusion:* Patients with atrial fibrillation at high risk ($>7\%$ per year) and low risk ($<3\%$ per year) for thromboembolism can be identified by readily available clinical variables.

26 Do you think the authors' abstract is a reasonable summary of the paper?

_____

_____

27 What questions do you think remain unanswered by this paper?

_____

_____

_____

28

a Does this paper apply to your original clinical problem?

_____

_____

b   On balance, can you use these results to answer the question
     in the clinical scenario?

_____

_____

_____

_____

_____

_____

Title

Predictors of Thromboembolism in Atrial Fibrillation: I. Clinical Features of Patients at Risk

The Stroke Prevention in Atrial Fibrillation Investigators

Annals of Internal Medicine. 1992; **116:** 1–5.

APPENDIX

The Stroke Prevention in Atrial Fibrillation Investigators are the following (centers are listed in order of the number of patients enrolled):

Clinical Centers

David C. Anderson, MD; Richard W. Asinger, MD; Susan M. Newburg, RN, BSN; Cheryl C. Farmer, RN, MA; K. Wang, MD; Scott R. Bundlie, MD; Richard L. Koller, MD; Waclav M. Jagiella, MD; Susan Kreher, MD; Charles R. Jorgensen, MD; Scott W. Sharkey, MD: Hennepin County Medical Center, Minneapolis and Abbott Northwestern Hospital, Minneapolis, Minnesota; Greg C. Flaker, MD; Richard Webel, MD; Barbie Nolte, RN, BSN; Pat Stevenson, LPN; John Byer, MD; William Wright, MD: The University of Missouri-Columbia; James H. Chesebro, MD; David O. Wiebers, MD; Anne E. Holland, RN, BSN; Diane M. Miller, LPN; William T. Bardsley, MD; Scott C. Litin, MD; Irene Meissner, MD; Douglas M. Zerbe, MD: Mayo Clinic and Mayo Foundation, Rochester, Minnesota; John H. McAnulty, MD; Christy Marchant, RN. MBA; Bruce M. Coull, MD: Oregon Health Sciences University; George Feldman, MD; Arthur Hayward, MD; Elizabeth Gandara, RN; Kate MacMillan, RN, BSN; Nathan Blank, MD: Kaiser Permanente, Portland, Oregon; Anne D. Leonard, RN, BSN; Merrill C. Kanter, MD; Laura M. Isensee, MD; Elia S. Quiroga, LVN; Charles H. Presti, MD; Charles H. Tegeler, MD: University of Texas Health Science Center at San Antonio and Audie L. Murphy Veterans Hospital; William R. Logan, MD; William P. Hamilton, MD; Barbara J. Green, MD; Rebecca S. Bacon, RN, BSN: St John's Mercy Medical Center, St Louis, Missouri; Robert M. Redd, MD; Dorothy J. Cadell, RN; Camilo R. Gomez, MD; Denise L. Janoski, MD; Arthur J. Labovitz, MD: St Louis University Medical Center; Roger E. Kelley, MD; Robert Chahine, MD; Lilian Cristo, RN; Maite Palermo, RN, BSN: Odalys Perez, RN, BSN: University Miami School of Medicine; Williams M. Feinberg, MD; Brenda K. Vold, RN, BSN; Karl B. Kern, MD; Christopher Appleton, MD: The University of Arizona College of Medicine; Vincent T. Miller, MD; Connie J. Hockersmith, RN; Bruce A. Cohen, MD; Gary J. Martin, MD; Alan J. Pawlow, MD: Northwestern University Medical School, Chicago, Illinois; Jonathan L. Halperin, MD; Elizabeth B. Rothlauf, RN; Jesse M. Weinberger, MD; Martin E. Goldman, MD; Valentin Fuster, MD: Mount Sinai Medical Center, New York, New York; Howard C. Dittrich, MD; John F. Rothrock, MD; Carol Hagenhoff, RN, MPH: University of California San Diego Medical Center; Cathy M. Helgason, MD; George T. Kondos, MD; Julie Hoff, RN, MPH; Lisa Kaufmann, RN, BSN; R. R. Rabjohns, MD; R. P. McRae, MD; J. Ghali, MD: University of Illinois College of Medicine at Chicago and Peoria; Harold P. Adams Jr., MD; Ernest O. Theilen, MD; José Biller, MD; Donald D. Brown, MD; Ellis Eugene Marsh III, MD; Sara

J. Sirna, MD; Victoria L. Mitchell, RN: University of Iowa College of Medicine; Robert M. Rothbart, MD; Gretchen H. Bailey, RN; Carolyn Burkhardt, MD: University of Colorado School of Medicine; Joseph L. Blackshear, MD; Lori Weaver, RN; Gary Lee, MD; Gary Lane, MD; Frank Rubino, MD; Robert Safford, MD: Mayo Clinic, Jacksonville, Florida; Richard A. Kronmal, Ph.D., University of Washington, Seattle, Washington; Ruth McBride; Marion W. Athearn, MS; Lesly A. Pearce, MS; Elaine Nasco: Statistics and Epidemiology Research Corporation; Statistical Coordinating Center; Robert G. Hart, MD; Carla P. Sherman, RN, BSN; David G. Sherman, MD; Robert L. Talbert, PharmD.; Tina L. Dacy; Patricia A. Heberling: Clinical Coordinating Center, University of Texas Health Science Center at San Antonio.

Safety Monitoring Committee

Theodore Colton, ScD, Boston University; David E. Levy, MD, Cornell University (New York); James D. Marsh, MD, Harvard University; Boston, Massachusetts; K. M. A. Welch, MD, Henry Ford Hospital; Detroit, Michigan: John R. Marler, MD, Bethesda, Mary-and; Michael D. Walker, MD, Bethesda, Maryland: National Intitute of Neurological Disorders and Stroke.

Writing Committee

Richard W. Asinger, MD, Hennepin County Medical Center—Minneapolis; Robert G. Hart, MD, University of Texas—San Antonio; Cathy M. Helgason, MD, University of Illinois—Chicago and Peoria; William R. Logan, MD, St. John's Mercy Medical Center—St. Louis; Lesly A. Pearce, MS, Statistics and Epidemiology Research Corporation; David G. Sherman, MD, University of Texas—San Antonio.

Grant Support: By grant R01-NS-24224 from the Divison of Stroke and Trauma, National Institute of Neurological Disorders and Stroke.

Requests for Reprints: Lesly A. Pearce, MS, SPAF Statistical Coordinating Center, Statistics & Epidemiology Research Corporation, 1107 NE 45th Street, Suite 520, Seattle, WA 98105.

References

1. Wolf PA, Dawber TR, Thomas HE Jr, and Kannel WB. Epidemiologic assessment of chronic atrial fibrillation and risk of stroke. The Framingham Study. *Neurology* 1978; **28:** 973–7

2. Wolf PA, Abbott RD, and Kannel WB. Atrial fibrillation: a major contributor to stroke in the elderly. The Framingham Study. *Arch Intern Med* 1987; **147:** 1561–4

3. Rodstein M, Moise S, Neufeld R, Wolloch L, and Mulvihill M. Nonvalvular atrial fibrillation and strokes in the aged. *Journal of Insurance Medicine* 1989; **21:** 192–4

4. Halperin JL and Hart RG. Atrial fibrillation and stroke: new ideas, persisting dilemmas. *Stroke* 1988; **19:** 937–41

5. Stroke Prevention in Atrial Fibrillation Investigators. The Stroke Prevention in Atrial Fibrillation Study: final results. *Circulation* 1991; **84:** 527–39

6. Petersen P, Boysen G, Godtfredsen J, Andersen ED, and Andersen B. Placebo-controlled, randomised trial of warfarin and aspirin for prevention of thromboembolic complications in chronic atrial fibrillation. The Copenhagen AFASAK study. *Lancet* 1989; **1:** 175–9

7. Connolly SJ, Laupaucis A, Gent M, Roberts RS, Cairns JA, Joyner C, and CAFA Study Co-investigators. Canadian Atrial Fibrillation Anticoagulation (CAFA) Study. *J Am Coll Cardiol* 1991; **18:** 349–55

8. Kopecky SL, Gersh BJ, McGoon MD, Whisnant JP, Holmes DR Jr, Ilstrup DM, and Frye RL. The natural history of lone atrial fibrillation. A population-based study over three decades. *N Engl J Med* 1987; **317:** 669–74

9. Cerebral Embolism Task Force. Cardiogenic brain embolism. The second report of the Cerebral Embolism Task Force. *Arch Neurol* 1989; **46:** 727–43

10. The Boston Area Anticoagulation Trial for Atrial Fibrillation Investigators. The effect of low-dose warfarin on the risk of stroke in nonrheumatic atrial fibrillation. *N Engl J Med* 1990; **323:** 1501–11

11. The Stroke Prevention in Atrial Fibrillation Investigators. Design of a multicenter randomized trial for the Stroke Prevention in Atrial Fibrillation Study. *Stroke* 1990; **21:** 538–45

12. Aronow WS, Gutstein H, and Hsieh FY. Risk factors for thromboembolic stroke in elderly patients with chronic atrial fibrillation. *Am J Cardiol* 1989; **63:** 366–7

13. Petersen P, Kastrup J, Helweg-Larsen S, Boysen G, and Godtfedsen J. Risk factors for thromboembolic complications in chronic atrial fibrillation. *Arch Intern Med* 1990; **150:** 819–21

14. Flegel KM and Hanley J. Risk factors for stroke and other embolic events in patients with nonrheumatic atrial fibrillation. *Stroke* 1989; **20:** 1000–4

15. Cabin HS, Clubb KS, Hall C, Perlmutter RA, and Feinstein AR. Risk for systemic embolization of atrial fibrillation without mitral stenosis. *Am J Cardiol* 1990; **65:** 1112–6

16. Flegel KM, Shipley MJ, and Rose G. Risk of stroke in non-rheumatic atrial fibrillation. *Lancet* 1987; **1:** 526–9

17. Wiener I. Clinical and echocardiographic correlates of systemic embolization in nonrheumatic atrial fibrillation. *Am J Cardiol* 1987; **59:** 177

18. The Stroke Prevention in Atrial Fibrillation Investigators. Predictors of Thromboembolism in Atrial Fibrillation. II. Echocardiographic features of patients at risk. *Ann Intern Med* 1992; **116:** 6–12

19. Frome EL. The analysis of rates using Poisson regression models. *Biometrics* 1983; **39:** 665–74

20. Mehta CR, Patel NR, and Gray R. Computing an exact confidence interval for the common odds ratio in several 2×2 contingency tables. *J Am Statist Assoc* 1986; **80:** 969–72

21. Yusuf S, Wittes J, and Probstfield J. Evaluating effects of treatment in subgroups of patients within a clinical trial: the case of non-Q-wave myocardial infarction and beta blockers. *Am J Cardiol* 1990; **66:** 220–2

22. ISIS-2 Collaborative Group. Randomised trial of intravenous streptokinase, oral aspirin, both, or neither among 17,187 cases of suspected acute myocardial infarction. *Lancet* 1988; **2:** 349–60

23. Kannell WB, Abbott RD, Savage DD, and McNamara PM. Coronary heart disease and atrial fibrillation: The Framingham Study. *Am Heart J* 1983; **106:** 389–96

24. Kannell WB, Abbott RD, Savage DD, and McNamara PM. Epidemiologic features of chronic atrial fibrillation: The Framingham Study. *N Engl J Med* 1982; **306:** 1018–22

Complete the checklist

Now use the answers you have already given to complete the following checklist and assign a score to this paper. There is space for you to add comments about the paper before you decide your final score.

If you wish, you can compare your score and comments with ours, which you will find in the answers section at the back of the book. If you have access to the World Wide Web (via the Internet) you can also compare your scores with those of other readers of this book. Details of how to do this are given in Appendix III.

The checklist is designed to be generalized to other papers of this type. A full set of blank checklists is included at the end of the book, which can be copied for use with other papers.

RATING SCALE 5 FOR ARTICLE ON PROGNOSIS

		Ring the appropriate code			
		Yes	Unclear/ possibly	No	Not applicable
RESULTS					
1	Is the risk per unit time of the outcome event(s) given?	2	1	0	N/A
2	Is this risk of clinical importance?	2	1	0	N/A
3	Is the estimate of risk sufficiently precise?	2	1	0	N/A
VALIDITY					
Selection					
4	Was the phase of the disease well defined?	2	1	0	N/A
5	Were patients at a uniform point in this phase?	2	1	0	N/A
6	Was the referral pattern described?	2	1	0	N/A
Follow-up					
7	Was follow-up sufficiently complete (under 10% lost to follow-up)?	2	1	0	N/A
8	Were the outcome measurements objective?	2	1	0	N/A
9	Was outcome assessment 'blind'?	2	1	0	N/A
Statistical analysis					
10	Were additional prognostic factors allowed for?	2	1	0	N/A
11	Was validation of the prognostic factor(s) performed?	2	1	0	N/A
12	Were there reasonable numbers of events (10–20 events per prognostic factor)?	2	1	0	N/A
13	Were appropriate methods used?	2	1	0	N/A
14	Were 'unusual' methods justified?	2	1	0	N/A
UTILITY					
15	Do the results help me choose treatments?	2	1	0	N/A
16	Do the results help me reassure/counsel patients?	2	1	0	N/A

TOTAL (add ringed scores above): _____ **(A)**

No. of questions which actually applied to this article (maximum = 16): _____ **(B)**

Maximum possible score (2 × B): _____ **(C)**

OVERALL RATING (A/C expressed as a percentage): _____ %

COMMENTS:

EXERCISE 9 A systematic review

LEARNING OBJECTIVES

After working through this exercise, you should be able to:

A Recognize important elements particular to a systematic review.

B Summarize the evidence and conclusions of a paper which combines findings from other studies.

C Explain how the results in such a paper might apply to a clinical or policy problem.

KEY POINTS

- Individual studies may be inconclusive or contradict other findings.

- It may be possible to combine the findings from a number of studies into a single estimate of effect.

- Systematic reviews should be subject to the same standards as individual trials.

- Policy decisions, like clinical decisions, are helped by good evidence but are not determined by it.

CLINICAL RELEVANCE

- How can we get the most out of the studies we have?

- How can we summarize findings for clinicians and managers?

THE POLICY PROBLEM

You are a member of a multidisciplinary health service planning team. The responsibility of the team is to recommend how services should best be provided for patients who suffer a stroke. You are all agreed that, whenever possible, decisions should be informed by the best available research evidence, to ensure that the strategies you recommend are likely to be effective. In addition, because the available budget for local stroke services is necessarily limited, you are all agreed that your recommendations should aim to produce the greatest amount of health benefits for the resources available.

At the last meeting of the team, there was heated debate over whether patients who have only just suffered a stroke (i.e. have acute stroke) should continue to be treated on general medical wards, or whether you should recommend that a specialized acute stroke unit is set up to treat such patients. A consultant member of the team produced a study which seemed to show that mortality was lower for patients treated on stroke units. However, a physiotherapist cited two other studies, which had apparently been unable to show any definite benefit to stroke unit treatment.

How can you move beyond this apparently contradictory evidence and help the team to agree on a strategy?

A POSSIBLE SOLUTION

As an experienced practitioner of evidence based medicine, you turn to MEDLINE and search for a systematic review of stroke units. Your search yields a single citation, which looks promising. But can you explain its findings clearly to your colleagues – and does it help you in planning your local stroke service?

INTRODUCTION

Read the introduction to the paper, and answer the questions which follow it.

Because no routine effective treatment for acute ischaemic stroke is available,[1] good organisation of stroke services is especially important. Stroke intensive care units have not been found beneficial in reducing mortality or morbidity,[2] although the value of less intensive specialist stroke units remains in dispute. Stroke units may help to hasten recovery and reduce time in hospital,[3–5] but are not thought to influence survival or longterm functional outcome.[6,7] However, a well-designed evaluation of a small stroke unit[5] showed sustained improvements in survival and functional outcomes that were attributed to the combination of acute medical management and dedicated rehabilitation interventions. To evaluate whether more stroke patients survive if managed in specialist stroke units, we report results of a statistical overview of randomised trials of stroke management.

1 Can you concisely express the research question to be addressed in this paper, in terms of a patient population, an intervention and an outcome?

_____

_____

_____

2 What other possible outcomes do the authors mention?

_____

_____

_____

3   The authors have conducted a 'statistical overview' of existing randomized trials. What else might they have done to answer the research question they have set, and why do you think they have chosen this approach?

_____

_____

_____

_____

_____

_____

_____

METHODS

Now read the methods section, and answer the questions which follow.

We tried to identify all randomised trials that compared patient management within specialist stroke units with standard, non-specialist services available at the time of the study. The inclusion criteria, based on an earlier definition of a stroke unit,[6] were: randomised controlled trial of acute stroke patients; control group in general medical/neurology wards; and stroke unit that included a multidisciplinary team of specialists in the care of stroke patients. These criteria apply to a geographically defined stroke unit or a mobile stroke team.

We identified research reports of stroke management for the period up to January, 1993, in *Index Medicus,* MEDLINE (English and foreign language), conference abstracts, bibliographies from major articles, textbooks, and reviews. We also tried to find unpublished trials by discussions with colleagues and past investigators in stroke management, and by publicising our preliminary findings at national and international stroke conferences. Two investigators independently assessed reports to confirm eligibility criteria and results. Our analysis did not include 1 small randomised trial of a stroke intensive care unit[8] because of the limited details available. We also excluded several studies that compared physiotherapy techniques,[9] and studies that evaluated late rehabilitation interventions.[10–15]

The primary outcome was mortality within 17 weeks of a stroke (median follow-up 13 weeks, range 5–17 weeks). Mortality at final review (median follow-up 12 months, range 6–12 months) was also recorded. Details of the cause of death were not usually available. Functional outcomes could not be analysed because of the variety of outcome measures used.

Studies were analysed on an intention-to-treat basis. Patients who were lost to follow-up were assumed to be alive, but a minor bias in favour of patients in general wards may have been introduced because more of these were lost to follow-up. Standard methods of overview analysis[16] were used for the calculation of odds ratios (with 95% confidence intervals), and odds reduction (with standard deviation) of mortality for individual trials and combined data. Conventional two-sided p-values (2p) are used throughout.[16]

4   The subjects of this study are randomized trials, rather than
     individual patients. How did the authors identify the trials to
     be included?

     _____

     _____

     _____

5   What criteria did the authors use in deciding which of the
     studies they found should be included in their review?

     _____

     _____

     _____

     _____

     _____

6   Do you think these criteria are sufficiently precise? Why?

     _____

     _____

     _____

     _____

     _____

     _____

     _____

     _____

7   Do you think it likely that the search described identified all
     important trials which would meet the inclusion criteria?

     _____

     _____

     _____

     _____

     _____

8   Why did the investigators try to find unpublished trials?

     _____

     _____

     _____

     _____

     _____

9   Did the investigators make sure all the studies included were
     well designed and carried out?

     _____

     _____

     _____

Study/location	Intervention	Time to entry to stroke unit (days)	Time in stroke unit (weeks)	No of patients
Feldman[17]/USA	Formal rehabilitation	<60	NK	82
Peacock[18]/USA	Intensive rehabilitation	<14	NK	52
Garraway[3]/Scotland	Stroke rehabilitation ward	<7	<16	311
Hamrin[23]/Sweden*	Systematic early active rehabilitation	<3	<4	112
Stevens[19]/England	Stroke rehabilitation ward	<21	NL	228
Wood-Dauphinee[20]/Canada	Mobile stroke team	<7	<5	126
Sivenius[21]/Finland	Intensive rehabilitation	<7	NL	95
Strand[25]/Sweden*	Non-intensive stroke unit	<7	NL	293
Indredavik[5]/Norway	Acute & rehabilitation stroke unit	<7	<6	220
Aitken[22]/England	Geriatric rehabilitation ward	<3	NL	67

Table 1 Details of published randomised trials of stroke unit care

* Informally randomised trials. NK = time in stroke unit not known, NL = time in stroke unit not limited.

10 The authors analysed study results on an 'intention-to-treat' basis. What is meant by this term? Do you think it was appropriate for this purpose?

_____

_____

_____

_____

_____

RESULTS OF THE SEARCH FOR TRIALS

The authors report the result of their search for trials as follows:

10 published trials were identified that used some form of randomisation and compared the intervention group with routine non-specialist care in general medical or neurology wards (Table 1). We were also told of a further 4 trials (based in Kent and Nottingham in the UK, Helsinki in Finland, and in Perth, Australia) for which final details were not yet available. 8 of the available trials[3–5,17–22] used a formal procedure with sealed envelopes or random numbers. In 2 trials, allocation was by an informal randomisation procedure: strict admission rota,[23,24] or 'first-come, first-served' policy for the stroke unit with excess patients going to general medical wards.[25] These 2 trials were evaluated separately to exclude any significant bias in the conclusions.

5 of the trials selected evaluated the impact of a geographically discrete stroke ward[3-5,19,25] or mobile stroke team.[20] The remainder looked at different methods of providing a more intensive[18,21] or more comprehensive[17,22-24] package of stroke rehabilitation. These trials were included in the analysis because the intervention group comprised a specialist team with an interest in stroke rehabilitation based at a separate location from the controls.

Study populations were all reported to be mixed with respect to sex and social background, and usually had a mean age of over 70 years. The same definition of stroke was used by all investigators—focal neurological deficit due to cerebrovascular disease excluding subarachnoid haemorrhage and subdural haematoma. The studies varied considerably in their selection criteria and in the proportion of eligible patients enrolled for randomisation.

The majority of reports[3,5,19,21,25] indicated that remedial therapy (physiotherapy, occupational therapy, speech therapy) was provided to a greater proportion of strike unit patients than controls. Stroke unit patients started remedial therapy earlier than controls in 3 studies.[3,5,25] The maximum duration of rehabilitation in the stroke unit varied from 5 weeks[20] to several months.[17,19,21,22,25]

The assessment of 2 studies was complicated by novel medical practices within the stroke units. Strand et al[25] included 21 of 110 patients in a haemodilution trial, but this is unlikely to have introduced important bias because haemodilution has not been shown to have any significant treatment effect.[26] Indredavik et al[5] used low-dose heparin in stroke unit patients with extensive paresis.

Mortality details were published for all except 2 reports;[21,22] unpublished results were provided by these authors. Minor omissions of data occurred in 4 studies[3,4,18,19,25] because of withdrawal of patients or loss to follow-up (0 for stroke unit patients and 11 for controls at initial review; 6 for stroke unit and 14 for controls at final review). The remaining studies either reported no withdrawals[17,20,24] or provided sufficient details to allow an 'intention-to-treat' analysis.[5]

11   **What further information is now available about the quality and comparability of the trials?**

_____

_____

_____

_____

_____

_____

_____

12   In general terms, how might you combine the evidence from each of these ten trials so that you could decide whether stroke units are beneficial?

_____

_____

_____

_____

_____

_____

_____

_____

_____

_____

RESULTS OF THE META-ANALYSIS OF TRIALS

This is how the results of the meta-analysis are presented:

Management of stroke patients within a stroke unit was associated with lower mortality rates than controls at both initial (Figure 1) and final (Figure 2) reviews. There was a 28% (SD 12, 2p < 0·01) reduction in the odds of death occurring in the first 17 weeks post-stroke (median follow-up 13 weeks, range 5–17) for patients in stroke units. This effect was sustained when mortality in the first year was recorded (median follow-up 12 months, range 6–12), with an odds reduction of death of 21% (SD 10, 2p < 0·05). Exclusion of trials with an informal randomisation procedure[23–25] resulted in calculated reductions in mortality for patients in stroke units of 37% (SD 12, 2p < 0·01) at initial review and 25% (SD 12, 2p < 0·05) at final review. Similar trends in mortality reduction were observed in each subgroup of trials (stroke ward, stroke team, intensive rehabilitation, comprehensive rehabilitation). Chi-square tests for heterogeneity between trials were non-significant for results at both initial (χ^2 5·5, 8 degrees of freedom) and final review (χ^2 1·93, 7 df).

Statistical overviews are liable to distortion because of publication bias. The reliability of the overview conclusions was estimated by calculating how many unpublished neutral studies would be required to alter our conclusions.[27] If we assume a mortality rate of 25%, then all our conclusions on survival benefit of a stroke unit would be refuted by several trials (1600 patients in total) that showed neutral results (odds ratio 1·0). If all the identified unpublished trials in progress were to produce neutral results, our conclusions would not be substantially altered.

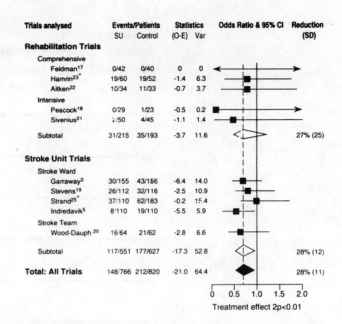

Figure 1 Initial mortality after stroke: stroke unit (SU) *vs* general wards (control).
* Informally randomised trials. O–E indicates observed minus expected number of events in treatment (SU) group; var denotes variance. ■ = odds ratio of death in stroke unit group *vs* in general wards for each trial with its 95% CI (horizontal line); ◇ = overview of trial results and 95% CI; ◆ = total for all trials. Reduction = reduction in overall mortality for these trials. Broken vertical line is odds ratio for all available trials.

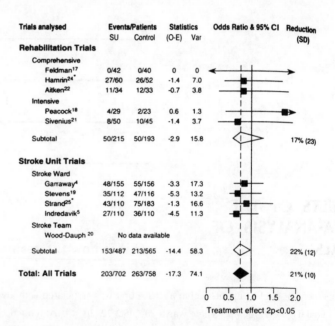

Figure 2 Mortality within 1 year of a stroke: stroke unit (SU) *vs* general wards (control). See Figure 1 for explanation of symbols.

Box 9.1: Reviews, systematic reviews and meta-analysis

The commonest form in which results from more than one study are combined is in a narrative **review**. Reviews may be long or short, comprehensive or selective, broad or narrow in scope. For example, a journal editorial might be a short, selective narrowly focused review of five or ten papers on a given topic. By contrast, a book chapter might attempt a wide-ranging, complete and in-depth review of a topic, with hundreds of studies included.

In general, such reviews rely on expert knowledge and understanding of an area to pick out important findings, combine evidence in interesting ways, and put forward a particular line of thought. There is no guarantee in such a process that the selection of evidence and the emphasis placed on different findings will be objective, or would be reproduced in quite the same way by a different expert in the field.

A **systematic review** (sometimes termed an 'overview') is an attempt to minimize the element of arbitrariness in an overview by making explicit the review process so that, in principle, another reviewer with access to the same resources could undertake the review and reach broadly the same conclusions. This requires that a systematic review has a clear and stated objective, an explicit and comprehensive search strategy for evidence, an explicit system for grading the quality of the evidence obtained, and a clear way of combining the evidence from individual studies to reach conclusions. It is almost as if a systematic review is a study which takes research studies as its subjects, instead of patients.

In many systematic reviews, there will be no sensible way to combine the evidence from different studies numerically, because the populations, interventions or outcome measures of the various studies are different. Nonetheless, it will be possible to explicitly grade the quality of the studies, in much the same way as has been taught in this book, so that the reviewer can weigh up the overall balance of evidence in reaching conclusions.

Sometimes it will be possible to combine the results of studies numerically, and this is termed **meta-analysis**. In some cases, a meta-analysis will be done using the aggregate results reported from each study, while in others the individual patient data will be re-analysed as if all the patients from different trials had entered a single trial together. The relative merits of these approaches are discussed in Box 9.2. Meta-analysis is a powerful technique which may allow important clinical questions to be answered by combining studies which, individually, have failed to provide a clear answer.

Where to find out more

Chalmers I and Altman DG. *Systematic Reviews*. BMJ Publishing Group, London, 1995
Thompson SG and Pocock SJ. Can meta-analysis be trusted? *Lancet* 1991; **338:** 1127–1130

Box 9.2: Aggregate analysis versus individual patient analysis

When meta-analyses are based on published results, these have to be pooled in some way. Typically the results are expressed as relative risks, risk differences or odds ratios. Statistical methods exist for pooling these values (essentially by averaging them).

A meta-analysis can be thought of, in a sense, as a substitute for a multi-centre randomized controlled trial. But in such a trial *individual* patient records would be analysed, with some adjustment for the centre (e.g. hospital) from which the record originated. Likewise, meta-analyses can be improved if individual patient records are made available: material may be more accurate, better comparability of patient groups may be achieved, and records may be updated. More powerful analyses are also possible.

It is not surprising to find that the results of meta-analyses based on individual patient data may differ considerably from those based on analyses of published results in which individual records have already been aggregated. In addition, some outcome measures, such as 'times to event' data (needed in survival analyses for prognostic and clinical trial studies), cannot be reliably calculated from aggregate data.

Where to find out more

Chalmers I and Altman DG. *Systematic Reviews*. BMJ Publishing Group, London, 1995
Stewart LA and Parmar MKB. Meta-analysis of the literature or of individual patient data: is there a difference? *Lancet* 1993; **341**: 418–422

---

13   The results of each individual trial, and of all ten trials combined using a meta-analytical technique, are presented in terms of an odds ratio with a 95% confidence interval (CI).

In order to be reasonably sure that treatment in a stroke unit reduces mortality, what do we require of the odds ratio and its 95% CI?

_____

_____

_____

_____

_____

_____

_____

14   Looking at Figures 1 and 2, do you think it would have been possible, without performing a meta-analysis, to reach a firm conclusion about the effects of stroke unit care on:

a   Initial mortality?

_____

_____

_____

_____

_____

b   Mortality within 1 year?

_____

_____

_____

_____

15   The result of statistically combining all of the trial results into a single estimate is shown in each figure by a black diamond.

Do the results given in the text match the results presented in the figures? Overall, what is the effect of stroke unit care on initial and longer term mortality?

_____

_____

_____

_____

16   How do the authors take account of the unknown results of trials currently in progress?

_____

_____

_____

_____

_____

_____

DISCUSSION   Now read the discussion section of the paper.

The main consideration of our overview was the way in which patient care is organised in the initial period after a stroke. We used a broad definition of a stroke unit and selected a heterogeneous group of trials, all of which examined stroke management in a unit with a specialist interest or expertise, irrespective of details of the management provided. A case could be made for the inclusion of only trials that aimed to evaluate a discrete stroke ward or team.[3-5,19,20,25] However, we felt that this would exclude several trials[17,18,21-24] in which the definition of a stroke unit[6] was fulfilled, although the aim of the study was to evaluate an aspect of rehabilitation. As shown by the homogeneity of mortality results from different trials, no individual component of the services given had any overwhelming influence on the conclusions. All trials involved a specialist multidisciplinary team that provided continuity of care during the first few weeks of illness.

The quality of publications included in an overview clearly influences the reliability of its conclusions. Although 2 of the studies[23-25] were randomised informally, our conclusions were confirmed by data from studies with formal randomisation procedures.[3-5,17-22] The small number of patients lost to follow-up was insufficient to bias our conclusions. In one trial, the randomisation procedure,[19] resulted in a greater proportion of patients with poor prognosis (initially reduced consciousness) in the control group. However, reanalysis of these results, such that only fully conscious patients are included, provides very similar conclusions.

We chose to express outcomes in terms of mortality because mortality is not subject to observer bias. Early mortality (within 6 months) has been the most common outcome in trials of acute stroke therapies.[26,28-30] We also include results at final review to ensure that any improvements were sustained. Although the reductions in mortality that we ascribe to stroke unit care are relatively imprecise, it should be noted that only two other interventions (calcium antagonists and haemodilution) have been subject to a greater number of trials.[1] None of the acute stroke therapies subjected to formal overview (calcium antagonists,[28] haemodilution,[26] heparin,[29] and glycerol[30]) have had any significant effect on mortality.

A stroke treatment should reduce morbidity as well as mortality. There was no evidence in the trials we reviewed that morbidity was increased by improved survival. All 10 studies recorded some aspect of functional outcome. 9 reported functional gains[3 5,17 22,25] in patients in stroke units; 4 achieved statistical significance.[3-5,21,25] Hamrin[23,24] described very similar outcomes in both groups. No investigator reported poorer functional outcomes among patients in stroke units. A more detailed analysis of functional outcomes was limited by the lack of consistent recording of outcome between trials.

Stroke units provide complex and varied interventions including medical, nursing, and remedial therapy. Our overview does not indicate which interventions improve survival. Indredavik et al,[5] whose study provides the most compelling evidence in favour of stroke units, hypothesised that the benefits were due to an integrated approach linking acute treatment with early mobilisation and rehabilitation. They emphasised the importance of early rehabilitation (usually within 24 hours) and of active participation of both patient and family. Although the medical interventions used by investigators in our overview may have influenced outcomes, the homogeneity of effect indicates a basic common factor in stroke unit practice.

In conclusion, our statistical overview of published stroke unit trials indicates that management in these units is associated with sustained improvements in survival. Although the important aspects of stroke unit management could not be identified, we believe that there is sufficient evidence to recommend better organised specialist stroke services that would, in turn, facilitate studies of specific components of stroke unit practice.

17   How have the investigators dealt with trials which have methodological weaknesses?

_____

_____

_____

_____

_____

_____

18   Are you concerned that stroke unit care might result in better survival rates, but more severe disability in those who do survive?

_____

_____

_____

_____

Box 9.3: Intention to treat analysis

In practice, some patients may not stay with the treatment they were originally given. For example patients receiving the 'new' treatment may be moved to the 'standard practice' group as a result of side-effects or lack of response (see diagram).

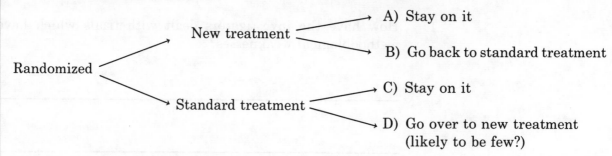

In the absence of any bias, random allocation guarantees that if there is *really* no difference between the treatments to which patients were assigned, the 'effect' *observed* in a given trial is a matter of chance. Analysing the results according to the *treatment actually received* removes this guarantee, and strictly speaking invalidates the basis for statistical analysis. In addition bias is very likely: the original balance of extraneous variables resulting from randomization will be lost, and because the patients are likely to drop out of the new treatment group because of adverse effects, the apparent effect is likely to be over-optimistic.

Analysis by 'intention to treat' keeps the patients in the original groups for statistical analysis, whether or not they actually completed (or even received) the treatment to which they were allocated, i.e. comparing groups A + B versus groups C + D, and therefore gives a pragmatic estimate of the value of the new treatment.

Studies that concentrate on clinical efficacy (simply establishing that the new treatment can work better than the standard in ideal circumstances) do compare group A versus group C, but special efforts have to be made to minimize the size of groups B and D, and this is generally possible only in relatively small trials.

Where to find out more

Newell DJ. Intention to treat analysis: implications for quantitative and qualitative research. *Int J Epidemiol* 1992; **21**: 837–841

19   The authors argue that 'the homogeneity of effect indicates a basic common factor in stroke unit practice'. What does this statement mean, and do you agree with it?

Does the paper help you with your problem?

20   What is the main conclusion of the paper?

_____

_____

21   Is this main conclusion supported by the evidence presented?

_____

_____

_____

22   What factors would you want to consider in deciding whether the findings of the paper apply to your own situation?

_____

_____

_____

_____

23   Has this paper helped you solve the problem you started with?

_____

_____

_____

_____

_____

_____

Abstract

Finally, the authors' summary of their findings is reproduced below.

Management of stroke patients in specialist stroke units hastens recovery but is not believed to influence mortality. We did a statistical overview of randomised controlled trials reported between 1962 and 1993 in which the management of stroke patients in a specialist unit was compared with that in general wards.

We identified 10 trials, 8 of which used a strict radomisation procedure. 1586 stroke patients were included; 766 were allocated to a stroke unit and 820 to general wards. The odds ratio (stroke unit *vs* general wards) for mortality within the first 4 months (median follow-up 3 months) after the stroke was 0·72 (95% CI 0·56–0·92), consistent with a reduction in mortality of 28% (2p < 0·01). This reduction persisted (odds ratio 0·79, 95% CI 0·63–0·99, 2p < 0·05) when calculated for mortality during the first 12 months. The findings were not significantly altered if the analysis was limited to studies that used a formal randomisation procedure.

We conclude that management of stroke patients in a stroke unit is associated with a sustained reduction in mortality.

Title

Do stroke units save lives?   Peter Langhorne, Brian O Williams, William Gilchrist, Kate Howie

Lancet 1993; **342:** 395–98.

We thank Dr M S Dennis, Dr P A G Sandercock, Prof C P Warlow, and Mr J Slattery for their assistance in the preparation of this report. Dr J Sivenius, Dr H Rogers, and Prof W M Garraway kindly supplied unpublished data. Dr K Asplund, Dr J McDonald, and Dr S Sanders gave helpful comments.

Department of Geriatric Medicine, Gartnavel General Hospital, Glasgow, UK (P Langhorne MRCP, B O Williams FRCP, W Gilchrist MRCP); *and University Department of Medicine, Gardiner Institute, Western Infirmary, Glasgow* (K Howie BSc)
Correspondence to: Dr Peter Langhorne, Department of Clinical Neurosciences, Western General Hospital, Edinburgh EH4 2XU, UK.

References

1. Sandercock P and Willems H. Medical treatment of acute ischaemic stroke. *Lancet* 1992; **339:** 537–39

2. Millikan CH. Stroke intensive care units: objectives and results. *Stroke* 1979; **10:** 235–37

3. Garraway WM, Akhtar AJ, Hockey L, and Prescott RJ. Management of acute stroke in the elderly: preliminary results of a controlled trial. *BMJ* 1980; **280:** 1040–44

4. Garraway WM, Akhtar AJ, Hockey L, and Prescott RJ. Management of acute stroke in the elderly: follow-up of a controlled trial. *BMJ* 1980; **281:** 827–29

5. Indredavik B, Bakke F, Solberg R, Rokseth R, Haahein LL, and Holme I. Benefit of stroke unit: a randomised controlled trial. *Stroke* 1991; **22:** 1026–31

6. Garraway WM. Stroke rehabilitation units: concepts, evaluation, and unresolved issues. *Stroke* 1985; **16:** 178–81

7. Ebrahim S. Clinical epidemiology of stroke. Oxford: Oxford University Press (Medical Publications), 1990

8. Erila T and Ilmavirta M. Does an intensive-care stroke unit reduce the early case-fatality rate of ischaemic stroke? *Stroke* 1990; **21:** 8 (suppl I): 153

9. de Pedro-Cuesta J, Widen-Holmquist L, and Bach-y-Rita P. Evaluation of stroke rehabilitation by randomised controlled studies: a review. *Acta Neurol Scand* 1992; **86:** 433–39

10. Smith DS, Goldenberg E, Ashburn A, et al. Remedial therapy after stroke: a randomised controlled trial. *BMJ* 1981; **282:** 517–20

11. Wade DT, Langton-Hewer R, Skilbeck CE, Bainton D, and Burns-Cox C. Controlled trial of a home-care service for acute stroke patients. *Lancet* 1985; **i:** 323–26

12. Young JB and Forster A. The Bradford community stroke trial: results at six months. *BMJ* 1992; **304:** 1085–89

13. Sunderland A, Tinson DJ, Bradley EL, Fletcher D, Langton Hewer R, and Wade DT. Enhanced physical therapy improves recovery of arm function after stroke: a randomised controlled trial. *J Neurol Neurosurg Psychiatry* 1992; **55:** 530–35

14. Wade DT, Collen FM, Robb GF, and Warlow CP. Physiotherapy intervention late after stroke and mobility. *BMJ* 1992; **304:** 609–13

15. Gordon EE and Kohn KH. Evaluation of rehabilitation methods in the hemiplegic patient. *J Chron Dis* 1966; **19**: 3–16

16. Peto R. Why do we need systematic overviews of randomised trials? *Stat Med* 1987; **6**: 233–40

17. Feldman DJ, Lee PR, Unterecker J, Lloyd K, Rusk HA, and Toole A. A comparison of functionally orientated medical care and formal rehabilitation in the management of patients with hemiplegia due to cerebrovascular disease. *J Chron Dis* 1962; **15**: 297–310

18. Peacock PB, Riley CHP, Lampton TD, Raffel SS, and Walker JS. The Birmingham stroke, epidemiology and rehabilitation study. In: Stewart GT, ed. Trends in epidemiology. Springfield, Illinois: Thomas, 1972: 231–345

19. Stevens RS, Ambler NR, and Warren MD. A randomised controlled trial of a stroke rehabilitation ward. *Age Ageing* 1984; **13**: 65–75

20. Wood-Dauphinee S, Shapiro S, Bass E, et al. A randomised trial of team care following stroke. *Stroke* 1984; **5**: 864–72

21. Sivenius J, Pyorala K, Heinonen OP, Salonen JT, and Riekkinen P. The significance of intensity of rehabilitation after stroke—a controlled trial. *Stroke* 1985; **16**: 928–31

22. Aitken PD, Rodgers H, French JM, Bates D, and James OFW. General medical or geriatric unit care for acute stroke? a controlled trial. *Age Ageing* 1993; **22** (suppl 2): 4–5

23. Hamrin E. Early activation after stroke: does it make a difference? *Scand J Rehabil Med* 1982; **14**: 101–09

24. Hamrin E. One year after stroke: a follow-up of an experimental study. *Scand J Rehabil Med* 1982; **14**: 111–16

25. Strand T, Asplund K, Eriksson S, Hagg E, Lithner F, and Wester PO. A non-intensive stroke unit reduces functional disability and the need for long-term hospitalisation. *Stroke* 1985; **16**: 29–34

26. Asplund K. Haemodilution in acute stroke. *Cerebrovasc Dis* 1991; **1** (suppl 1): 129–38

27. Rosenthal R. The 'file drawer problem' and tolerance for null results. *Psychol Bull* 1979; **86**: 638–41

28. Gelmers HJ and Hennerici M. Effect of nimodipine on acute ischaemic stroke: pooled results from five randomised trials. *Stroke* 1990; **21** (suppl IV): IV 81–84

29. Sandercock PAG, van den Belt AGM, Lindley RI, and Slattery J. Antithrombotic therapy in acute ischaemic stroke: an overview of the randomised trials. *J Neurol Neurosurg Psychiatry* 1993; **56**: 17–25

30. Rogvi-Hansen B and Boysen G. Intravenous glycerol treatment of acute stroke—a statistical overview. *Cerebrovasc Dis* 1992; **2**: 11–13

Complete the checklist

Now use the answers you have already given to complete the following checklist and assign a score to this paper. There is space for you to add comments about the paper before you decide your final score.

If you wish, you can compare your score and comments with ours, which you will find in the answers section at the back of the book. If you have access to the World Wide Web (via the Internet) you can also compare your scores with those of other readers of this book. Details of how to do this are given in Appendix III.

The checklist is designed to be generalized to other papers of this type. A full set of blank checklists is included at the end of the book, which can be copied for use with other papers.

RATING SCALE 6 FOR OVERVIEW ARTICLE

		Ring the appropriate code			
		Yes	Unclear/ possibly	No	Not applicable
RESULTS					
1	Is a summary estimate of association (e.g. odds ratio, relative risk or risk difference) given?	2	1	0	N/A
2	Is this association of clinical importance?	2	1	0	N/A
3	Is the estimate of risk (or relative risk) sufficiently precise?	2	1	0	N/A
VALIDITY					
Selection					
4	Were inclusion criteria for the studies well defined?	2	1	0	N/A
5	Was a well-posed question addressed?	2	1	0	N/A
6	Were convincing efforts made to find all relevant studies?	2	1	0	N/A
7	Was the quality of the studies assessed?	2	1	0	N/A
Statistical analysis					
8	Was the quality of the studies allowed for in the analysis?	2	1	0	N/A
9	Was the quality assessment reproducible?	2	1	0	N/A
10	Was the analysis based on individual patient data?	2	1	0	N/A
11	Were results from each study similar enough to be pooled?	2	1	0	N/A
12	Were sources of variability identified?	2	1	0	N/A
UTILITY					
13	Do the results help me choose a treatment?	2	1	0	N/A
14	Were all clinically important outcomes considered?	2	1	0	N/A

TOTAL (add ringed scores above): _____ **(A)**

No. of questions which actually applied to this article (maximum = 14): _____ **(B)**

Maximum possible score (2 × B): _____ **(C)**

OVERALL RATING (A/C expressed as a percentage): _____ %

COMMENTS:

Answers to Exercises

EXERCISE 1

1   *To check how well pathologists agree when diagnosing molar pregnancy using 'recognized' histological criteria.*

2   *Because if hydatidiform mole is present in products of conception, patients need to be treated, but a recurring problem is 'partial mole' in which fetal tissue is present as well, which can obscure the diagnosis.*

3   *From pathology files at Royal Preston Hospital (non-teaching) and Jessop Hospital (teaching).*

4   *It is not specified.*

5   *Again this is not specified.*

6   *It is hard to tell; they could well be typical of the patients seen in those particular hospitals, but differ from other hospitals, especially outside the UK. If the case-mix did differ from that of your patients then the results of the study may not directly apply to your own laboratory.*

7   *As a form of blinding, so that pathologists would not recognize cases from their own hospital. See Box 1.1.*

8   *To allow pathologists to forget their original diagnosis and prevent special attention being paid on the second occasion to slides found noteworthy on the first reading.*

9   *To ensure that the pathologists' diagnoses were made in a standard way, hopefully reducing the effect of variations in their training to date. This assumes that agreement on the histological features would potentially be better than for the final diagnosis. It certainly offers the opportunity to clarify areas of disagreement. As a general rule, it pays to distinguish observations from ensuing conclusions.*

10   *This is not specified in the text but is included in the abstract (!): seven consultant (specialist grade) pathologists – two specializing in gynaecological pathology and five general hospital consultant pathologists.*

11

  a   *By using the kappa statistic – denoted in the text by the Greek letter κ.*

  b   *By the percentage of agreement between two runs by the same pathologist.*

12 *The essential question is why they did not use kappa for intra-rater agreement as well as inter-rater agreement? We find this odd.*

13 *Presumably as 'type' illustrations of the three conditions under consideration. How they were chosen is not clear. It might have been better to display two examples of each condition, those that the raters agreed on least, and those for which agreement was greatest (according to original classification). This is part of the same message as question 9: standardized criteria help improve agreement. In other words, only expect agreement to be high if you have established standards!*

14 *Yes, you should be able to do so.*

15 *0.573. This is a fairly typical value for inter-rater agreement among histopathologists; for example, in one study, kappa for level of invasion of malignant melanoma was 0.59. By contrast, in another study kappa for tumour thickness was 0.88, supporting the use of tumour thickness rather than level of invasion as a prognostic indicator for melanoma. For other clinical examples see Koran LM. The reliability of clinical methods, data and judgements. N Engl J Med 1975; **292:** 642–646, 695–701.*

We can, of course, also apply kappa to within-observer (intra-rater) agreement, giving an index of self-consistency.

16

Intra-rater agreement for Observer A (counts of observations)

First reading	Second reading			Total
	Non-molar	Partial mole	Complete mole	
Non-molar	23	5	$A = 0$	28
Partial mole	$B = 1$	$C = 5$	$D = 2$	8
Complete mole	$E = 0$	$F = 0$	14	$G = 14$
Total	24	10	$H = 16$	$I = 50$

$P_o = 0.84$ (given in Table 5 as a percentage), $P_e = 0.3906$, kappa = 0.74.

17 *0.57–0.90. Using Everitts formula they are 0.53–0.94.*

18

a *Complete mole can be distinguished from non-molar pregnancy.*

b *It can be hard to distinguish non-molar pregnancy from partial mole.*

c   *Pathologists were generally **self**-consistent, but agreed poorly with **each other**.*

d   *Other diagnostic tests might help, e.g. ploidy studies.*

19   *What about validating histology against ploidy? Was agreement better between the 'expert' pathologists? Was the Australian pathologist different from the others? Would agreement be better with special training? What would agreement be like on the individual diagnostic categories? The authors did not describe the conditions under which the study was carried out (e.g. were slides inserted into routine reporting sessions? were participants told the proportions of each category to be expected?), nor whether any special training was provided (e.g. to make the diagnosis by reference to 'typical' pictures). These are points we picked up – you may have noted others.*

20   *Compare your abstract with that of the investigators.*

21

a   *There are some problems with the results: the authors did not present kappa for agreement of complete mole vs non-molar pregnancy, and the joint agreement of five pathologists was not corrected for chance. Confidence limits were not given.*

b   *There is the point mentioned earlier that the range of specialists is only given in the abstract; the authors also state that 'experts' agreed no better than the others, but we cannot verify this from the results given in the paper.*

22   *No, although one cannot tell very much just from one instance. One might expect better agreement among colleagues who have worked together for many years than from a random assortment of pathologists. Your colleagues could carry out an inter-observer agreement study to see whether their inter-rater kappa is comparable with that of this study; to improve agreement they could try to agree criteria for each diagnosis, maybe use some (semi)quantitative measurements – all with the aim of standardizing diagnostic conditions and reducing subjectivity.*

Checklist score: Our score was 66%

EXERCISE 2

1   *In a population of primary care patients (the patient type), can the CAGE questionnaire (the measurement) distinguish patients with alcohol problems from those without (the outcome)?*

2   *To easily and quickly detect people who are likely to be abusing, or dependent on, alcohol.*

3   *(Reader to supply.)*

4   *It should identify a **high** percentage of those people who have problems, and have a **low** risk of falsely identifying people who do not have a problem.*

5   *If the response to any two or more questions is 'yes', the test is positive.*

6   *Compare the scores from a sample of alcoholics with the scores from a sample of non-alcoholics, to see whether they differ.*

7   *All the English-speaking patients over 18 attending the Medical College of Virginia's outpatient (ambulatory) medical clinic between October 1988 and February 1990.*

8   *Demographic information was collected using CIDI-SAM (the Composite International Diagnostic Interview–Substance Abuse Module).*

     Screening test information was collected using the CAGE score.

     Reference information on alcoholism was collected using the alcohol module of the Diagnostic Interview Schedule (DIS).

9   *Age and sex; alcohol diagnosis and symptoms; age at onset and most recent symptoms.*

10   *The DIS alcohol module, which the authors imply has good sensitivity, specificity and predictive ability.*

11   *Odds = p/(1 − p). In this case, p = 0.2, so odds = 0.2/(1 − 0.2) = 0.25.*

12   *Probability = odds/(1 + odds). In this case, odds = 0.6, so p = 0.6/(1 + 0.6) = 0.375.*

13   *821*

14   *76 men were social drinkers; 91 women were abstainers*

15   *63% of men (i.e. the 46% who showed dependence plus the 17% who showed abuse); 23% of women (i.e. 14% plus 9%); 36% of all subjects (i.e. 25% plus 11%)*

16   *From equation (2), prior odds = (prior probability)/(1 − prior probability). Without any other information about an individual, our best estimate of their prior probability is the prevalence of alcoholism in the population, in this case 63% of men. This is an extremely high estimate and may reflect a broad definition of 'alcohol abuse' used by the authors.*

     So: prior odds = 0.63/(1 − 0.63) = 1.703.

17   *The first column gives each possible CAGE score. For each possible score, the second and third columns show the number of alcoholic and non-alcoholic subjects in the study who gave that score on screening.*

18   *Total alcoholic subjects = 294. Total non-alcoholic subjects = 527.*

19   *Proportion with score of **exactly** 1: 45/294 = 15.3%. Proportion with score of **at least** 1: 261/294 = 88.8%.*

20   *Proportion correctly identified = (Number correctly identified as alcoholic)/(All who were alcoholic) = (86 + 74 + 56)/294/73.5%.*

21   *The ratio of subjects correctly identified as having the condition to **all** subjects with the condition is the **sensitivity** of the test.*

22   *Proportion correctly identified = (Number correctly identified as **not** alcoholic)/(All who were **not** alcoholic) = (428 + 54)/527 = 91.5%.*

23 *The ratio of subjects correctly identified as **not** having the condition to **all** subjects without the condition is the **specificity** of the test.*

24 *The probability that an **alcoholic** subject has a CAGE score of 3 is $74/294 = 25\%$.*

   *The probability that a **non-alcoholic** subject has a CAGE score of 3 is $10/527 = 1.9\%$.*

25 *The ratio of these probabilities is $25/1.9 = 13$, which agrees with the value given by the authors. Note that, in Table 2, the values of sensitivity and specificity given for each CAGE score result from that score being used as a cut-off value, so that all those with that score or above are deemed positive, and those with a lower score are deemed negative.*

26 *Your curve should look like the one presented by the authors!*

27 *Technically, the best choice is that which gives the maximum vertical distance between the observed ROC curve and the line which describes the results of a test which cannot distinguish between alcoholics and non-alcoholics at all. This is represented by a straight line joining the origin to the 100/100 point.*

   In this case, the best cut-off point is a score of one.

28 *There is no single correct answer to this. The score you choose will depend on how you weigh the importance of, on the one hand, missing people with alcoholism and, on the other, incorrectly suspecting people of having an alcohol problem when they do not. In other words, it depends how you judge the consequences of underdiagnosis or overdiagnosis.*

   For a different approach to this problem, look at the recursive partitioning technique used in Exercise 3.

29 *Yes. All the published studies seem to give similar curves, all of which allow a choice of threshold with a high true-positive rate and a low false-positive rate.*

30 *Each column corresponds to an estimated prior probability of alcoholism. There is a row for each possible CAGE score. Each figure in the table gives the posterior probability of alcoholism for a person with the prior probability at the top of the column and the CAGE score at the left of the row.*

   In this case, we imagine a patient with an estimated prior probability of 20%. When we administer the CAGE questions, the patient scores 3. Using the table, we find the value 76, meaning that the patient's posterior probability (i.e. their probability now, knowing their responses) is 76%.

31 *Your method here should be to begin by converting the prior probability to a prior odds. In this case, prior odds $= p/(1 - p)$ $= 0.36/0.64 = 0.563$. For each value of the CAGE score, you then calculate the posterior odds as prior odds × likelihood ratio, and convert each posterior odds back to a posterior probability. The next answer gives you a worked example.*

32   *We estimate prior probability = prevalence = 0.28 (although it is arguable that people attending the doctor would have a slightly higher prevalence than those who do not attend).*

So: prior odds = $p/(1 - p) = 0.28/0.72 = 0.388$.

Likelihood ratio for CAGE score 1 = 1.5 (from Table 2).

Posterior odds = prior odds × likelihood ratio = $0.388 \times 1.5 = 0.583$.

Posterior probability = odds/(1 + odds) = $0.583/1.583 = 0.368$, or 37%.

33   *Your answer will depend on how you weigh up the risks and benefits of these courses of action for the patient and for others. The greater the costs to the patient of the course of action, the more certain you would want to be that they have an alcohol problem. In that case, you might consider other diagnostic tests or an extended consultation before deciding.*

34   *They suggest using available prevalence data. This is reasonable if data are available for populations similar to your own.*

35   *They argue for using likelihood ratios, because each different score can then indicate a level of risk. If a single cut-off is used, then all scores below the cut-off give one level of risk, and all scores above it give another level.*

36   *That the CAGE score is a good way to screen for alcoholism.*

37   *Yes, the evidence is convincing in showing the discriminating ability of the test.*

38   *Would the questions used make sense to your patients, in view of possible age, gender or cultural differences? Would the likelihood ratios be the same in your own population?*

39   *Yes. It seems a quick, easy, cheap and apparently fairly accurate way to detect your patients who may have an alcohol problem.*

Checklist score: Our score was 78%

EXERCISE 3

1   *Using an algorithm based on simple body measurements, can we accurately identify high risk (low birthweight, preterm) babies in a developing country population of newborn infants?*

Population: newborn infants.

Measurement/test: the algorithm.

Outcome: classified as high or low risk.

2   *The group at highest risk of health problems is the LBW, preterm group. Term LBW infants are 'developmentally mature' and have a lower risk of problems.*

3   *Because if weighing is delayed for a few days, the baby's weight is likely to have fallen in any case, and will give a false impression of LBW status.*

4   *It should enable us to accurately assign infants to either high risk or low risk groups, using only simple measurements which would be feasible in a rural area.*

5   *Quick and cheap to carry out.*

   Acceptable to the local population (of mothers and babies).

   Easy for health workers to learn to perform and interpret.

   Unambiguous.

   Not painful or harmful to the baby.

   No expensive or hard to obtain equipment required.

6   *The subjects were 843 infants who were admitted to the nursery or neonatal care unit of the Tikur Anbessa Hospital, Addis Ababa, who were not ruled out by the exclusion criteria.*

7   *In order to develop the screening algorithm, the investigators needed to know the 'correct answer' for each baby. If gestational age was uncertain, then the investigators would not know whether, in fact, the baby should be identified as high or low risk.*

8   *Gestational age.*

   Birthweight.

   Neonatal chest, head and mid-arm circumferences.

   Length of baby.

9   *To avoid the nurses being influenced in any way in their measurements by prior knowledge of the risk status of the baby. This possibility is termed 'measurement bias'. (See Box 1.1 on blinding.)*

10 *In general, yes. A false-negative error occurs when a baby is judged to be low risk when in fact it is high risk. Such an error might mean that care which could reduce the risk of ill-health for the baby might not be provided. The baby might suffer as a result of this misclassification.*

   On the other hand, a false-positive error occurs when a baby which is, in reality, at low risk is judged to be at high risk. Extra care might then be provided. This is unlikely to disadvantage the baby, though of course it would be wasteful of resources. It might even mean that another baby, which could have benefited more, is denied care.

11

a   *50/1 implies that the error of misclassifying a preterm LBW baby as term or normal is 50 times more serious than misclassifying a normal baby as preterm or LBW.*

b   *1/1 implies that all misclassifications of babies are equally undesirable.*

c   *1/10 implies that the error of misclassifying a low risk baby as high risk is 10 times more serious than misclassifying a high risk baby as low risk.*

12   *A sensitivity analysis is a way of testing the importance of various assumptions you might make, by varying one assumption at a time to see how this affects the results.*

In this case, the importance of the assumption of a misclassification cost ratio of 10/1 is tested. This is done by assuming a range of alternative ratios and looking at how different the results turn out to be.

13   *One group – the training group – is used to develop the algorithm. The algorithm is developed using both the predictive measurements and the outcome we are trying to predict.*

The other group – the validation group – will be used to test how well the algorithm performs once it has been developed. In this group we will imagine that we do not already know the outcome, and try to predict it using the algorithm. Then we compare the predicted outcome with the actual outcome to see how many 'right answers' the algorithm was able to generate.

14   *The authors use each tree to allocate all the babies in the training set into high or low risk. Then they add up the misclassification costs for all the babies who have been wrongly allocated by that tree.*

Clearly, trees that do not perform so well will produce a high total misclassification cost compared to trees that are better able to correctly classify the babies.

15   *You would want the tree to be as simple as possible, so that health workers would find it easy to use. The fewer measurements required, the better.*

16   *First, the tree with the lowest misclassification cost is identified. This is the 'best' tree in terms of performance, but it may be a fairly complex tree. It would be a good idea to be able to pick a simpler tree if one were available which performed almost as well.*

Second, trees which perform almost as well as the best are identified. These are trees with a misclassification cost 'within one standard error' of the lowest cost. (Consult a statistical textbook for an explanation of standard error.)

Third, from the original tree and those trees which perform almost as well, the simplest is taken as the best tree.

17   *From Table 1: mean age 276 days, standard deviation 22.6 days.*

18   *From Table 1: in the training group, 10% were high risk (LBW and preterm), and in the validation group, 7%.*

19

Subject	Head circumference (cm)	Chest circumference (cm)	Risk category using Algorithm A	Risk category using Algorithm B
Baby A	27	29	High	High
Baby B	32	28	High	Low
Baby C	33	31	Low	Low
Baby D	30	27	High	High

20   *Only baby B in this case. In general, Algorithm A will only classify differently from Algorithm B when the head circumference is greater than 31 cm, but the chest circumference is less than or equal to 30 cm. In such a case, the simpler Algorithm B will classify as low risk, while the more complex Algorithm A will classify as high risk.*

21

a   *Babies A and D could still be classified as high risk.*

b   *Babies A, B and D could still be classified as high risk.*

22   *The fall in the ratio implies that we have become relatively less concerned about missing a high risk baby, and relatively more concerned not to misclassify a low risk baby as high risk. Under these conditions, we can see intuitively that we need make 'less effort' to spot the high risk babies, which is equivalent in this instance to dropping the second branching based on chest circumference.*

23   *This is roughly equivalent to saying that we are relatively far more concerned to correctly classify a high risk baby than a low risk baby – we do not want to miss a baby at high risk, and we do not mind saying a baby is high risk when it is not.*

The tree which results from such an assumption would probably not be very much more complex than those presented, and might well be simpler. The main difference would be that the 'branching values' would be much higher than those presented in the paper.

24

a   *The PPV is the probability that a baby classified as high risk by the algorithm really is high risk. A PPV of about 50% means that only half of the babies we classify as high risk actually are.*

b   *Unlike the sensitivity and specificity, which are properties of the algorithm (or test) itself, the PPV also depends on the prevalence in the population of the condition we are trying to detect. If the prevalence is low, as in this case, then even a good test/algorithm will have a low PPV.*

Note that, using the recursive partitioning method, the decision about the relative importance of sensitivity, specificity and PPV is made implicitly when the misclassification cost ratio is decided upon at the start.

25 *The representativeness of the study population.*

The possibility that the measurements used may change in the few days after birth.

The possibility that gestational age was not measured accurately.

26 *A common approach to this sort of problem is to try using a single attribute of the baby – perhaps just the length – as a screening test. However, such a simplified approach cannot combine the information from a number of different measurements to improve the ability of the test to predict babies at high risk.*

*A second approach is to mathematically combine the different attributes measured using the techniques of multiple regression or logistic regression. While these techniques are beyond the scope of this book, the essential purpose is to arrive at a formula of the form $y = \beta_1 x_1 + \beta_2 x_2 + \beta_3 x_3 + \ldots$ where y is the value we are trying to predict and x_1, x_2, x_3 are our measured attributes of individuals. Using this approach it would be possible to construct a formula which, given the measurements of one baby, gave us the **probability** of that baby being at high risk. The formula $\beta_1 x_1 + \beta_2 x_2 + \beta_3 x_3 + \ldots$ would be a predictive (or prognostic) index, and different cut-points could be defined with different levels of sensitivity and specificity (see also Box 7.3).*

*The method used in this paper is interesting because it **begins** with an explicit decision about the 'costs' of being wrong about an individual. In addition, it has the advantage that the eventual result is an algorithm which is simple to understand and to use, and easy to pass on to others. In use, no difficult calculations are required. The authors also point out that it may sometimes be possible to use an algorithm even if some information about a baby is missing, as indicated in question 21.*

It is debatable whether this method is more or less difficult to use in research terms than a multiple regression approach.

27 *Yes, they have demonstrated this conclusion convincingly.*

28 *Could the babies in your hospital have been included in this study? In general, yes, since they are all within a day old. You would be less confident about applying this algorithm if any of the babies are from multiple births or have congenital malformations, since such babies were explicitly excluded in the study.*

You would have to assume that the population of Ethiopian babies used to develop the algorithm was substantially similar to the population of Zimbabwean babies for whom you are caring.

29 *Yes. The village health worker can use Algorithm A to try to identify which, if any, of the babies born in the last 24 hours are at high risk and therefore need the special care cot. The algorithm is simple enough to write down and send back to the village health worker to use locally.*

Of course, you might discover that more than one of the babies is classified as 'high risk' by the algorithm, and if this was the case you would still have a problem in allocating the cot. You would then have to consider the needs of the new babies against the babies already in special care.

30 *Yes, the summary is an accurate and concise description of the evidence, which could also be used as it stands to communicate the results of the paper to field health workers.*

Checklist score: Our score was 78%

EXERCISE 4

1 *In women in general (the patient type), is the use of the oral contraceptive pill (OCP, the exposure) associated with any increase (or decrease) in the risk of fatal venous thromboembolism (the outcome)? Based on previous work, our presumption is that an increase is more likely than a decrease in risk.*

2 *They cite evidence that the increase in risk is related to the oestrogen dose. Because the doses of both oestrogen and progestogen in the OCP have fallen over recent years, it is possible that use of the OCP may now not be associated with an increase in thromboembolism risk. It is worth discovering whether or not this is true.*

3 *Possible study designs could include:*

Ecological: comparing population rates of thromboembolism and of OCP use in different places or at different times, to see whether they vary together.

Case-control: comparing the exposure history of a group of women who have suffered the outcome of interest (the cases) with a group who have not (the controls).

Cohort: following a group of women using the OCP and a group not using it, recording the outcomes of interest in each group over a period of time. If event rates are likely to be low (as here) this will require a large cohort followed for a long period.

*A **randomized controlled trial** might be neither practical nor ethical in this context. While in general it is unethical to randomize patients to an intervention for which there is evidence of harm, it might be ethical in this case if the choice is between the older treatment and a newer (lower risk) treatment. However, it might be impractical if women have a strong preference for one treatment choice, and the same considerations regarding the low event rates would apply as in the cohort design.*

4   *This is a case-control study. Study subjects are grouped according to whether they have suffered the outcome of interest (in this case, as having died from a venous thromboembolism). The exposure of each subject (case or control) to a range of possible risk factors of interest can then be measured and compared between the groups.*

5   *Yes, given the need to examine a range of possible causes. The rarity of the outcome may also be a consideration. Case-control studies are generally quicker and cheaper to conduct than cohort studies, and the difference in efficiency becomes greater the rarer the outcome of interest. With a rare outcome the odds ratio which the study estimates will be a good approximation to the relative risk (see Box 4.1).*

6   *Through the national death certification system, using relevant codes for cause of death. The criteria for diagnosing cases are well defined in the paper, and rely on the accuracy and consistency of death certification. Since these are sudden deaths in young women, they are likely to have been confirmed by post-mortem examination in the majority of cases.*

7   *Two controls were identified from the same GP's list as each case. It is important in a case-control study that controls are, in principle, from the same population as the cases. This has been achieved in this study by selecting cases from the same GP's list, and this may have the added benefit of reducing the possibility of bias due to differences in the quality of GP case notes.*

8   *For both cases and controls, the investigators asked the GP for:*

past medical history

drug history

menstrual status

obstetric history

contraceptive use

parity

height

weight

blood pressure

smoking habits

The investigators also tried to collect more detailed information on smoking through a postal questionnaire, without much success.

9   *Matching in a case-control study is used to try to eliminate potential confounders. For example, in this study the investigators suppose that the outcome and the exposures may both be related to age. By matching cases and controls of similar ages, they can avoid a spurious observed association due to the effect of age (see Box 4.2).*

10 *Cause of death not confirmed, resident for at least 1 month in an institution, pregnant within the 2 months prior to death, or death preceded by a life-threatening illness.*

11 *Cause of death not confirmed: to ensure that 'cases' really are cases.*

Resident for at least 1 month in an institution, pregnant within the 2 months prior to death, death preceded by a life-threatening illness: since these are all factors which in themselves might lead to an increased risk of thrombosis and lower rates of OCP use. They are therefore potential **confounders**, *eliminated in this case by a strategy of restriction (see Box 4.2).*

12 *Measurement was by interview with the GP. If the GPs are able to refer to accurate case notes then this method may be accurate and unbiased. If the GPs rely to some extent on their own memory or knowledge of their patients they may tend to over- or underestimate OCP use. They may also be subject to bias, since they are themselves aware which women are cases (since they have died) and which are controls. They may be more careful to look for a record of OCP use for the cases (see Box 4.3 on bias).*

Given the nature of the study, it would not have been possible to 'blind' the GPs to the outcome status of the subjects, though it may have been possible to use an independent assessor to extract information from the case notes.

13 *The odds ratio is 4.0. This implies that the odds of a woman* **with** *a previous history suffering a fatal thromboembolism are 4 times the odds for a woman* **without** *such a history, and is approximately the relative risk.*

The confidence interval is 1.4–11.5. Loosely speaking, we interpret this to mean that we can be 95% certain that the true value of the OR is somewhere between 1.4 and 11.5.

14 *The ascertainment of exposure (to operation/accident) here may be subject to recall bias if details of past operations or accidents were not always recorded in case notes.*

15 *In both groups about one third of women were non-users. Among the cases, a greater proportion were current users than among the controls.*

16 *Although the point estimate of the OR is 1.6, the true value may plausibly be as low as 0.7. Therefore, the study has not been able to show that OCP use is definitely associated with increased risk of fatal venous thromboembolism. Nor can the study rule out an effect of the OCP.*

It may be that if the sample sizes had been larger, the lower limit of the confidence interval would have exceeded 1, thus making us reasonably certain of an increased risk from OCP use.

17 *Yes, the conclusions seem suitably reserved given the analysis above.*

18   *This study only examined fatal cases of thromboembolism. There may be qualitative differences between the risk factors for fatal and non-fatal disease. Women who suffer a fatal episode may be different in some way from those who do not. The authors hint at this possibility in their final paragraph.*

19   *Would my patient have been eligible for the study? In the clinical situation described, the patient would have been in- cluded, so long as she did not meet any of the exclusions given in the answer to question 10.*

     Did my patient have any of the risk factors confirmed in this study (i.e. operation, accident and previous thrombotic disease)?

20   *Regrettably, no, since the paper was unable to reach a definite conclusion one way or the other. You might now widen your search to try to identify other relevant papers on this issue.*

21   *Yes. All the findings and conclusions given in the abstract are also present in the body of the paper.*

     Checklist score: Our median score was 56%
                     (range among us 51–61%)

EXERCISE 5

1

     Patient: Male in 50–64 year age group with inflammatory bowel disease.

     Intervention: Azathioprine treatment (any dose/route) com- pared to 'other treatments'.

     Outcome: Neoplasia.

     Question: If azathioprine is given to men aged 50–64 years with inflammatory bowel disease, is the risk of neoplasia in the bowel (or any related site) increased?

2   *Patient: Any age, sex, with inflammatory bowel disease.*

     Intervention: Standard dose of azathioprine.

     Outcome: Any subsequent malignant disorder (up to 29 years follow up: median 9 years).

     Question: Do patients with inflammatory bowel disease given a standard dose of azathioprine have a risk of subsequent malignant disease greater than that of ... (the comparison is unclear)?

3   *Paper is unfocused in terms of age/sex, but specifically con- siders malignant neoplasia. It is not clear whether it will compare rates between azathioprine-treated and untreated groups.*

4   *By a register of patients which had been maintained pros- pectively (i.e. added to at the time) at a single hospital.*

5   *From hospital case notes.*

6   *Hospital case notes for current patients; for other live patients: present hospital physician or referring or present GP; for untraceable patients: NHS Central Register.*

7   *Deaths from all causes and deaths from neoplasia (in people under 85 years only).*

8   *Both cohorts consist of patients suffering CEUC, but in one the patients have received treatment with azathioprine, and in the other they have not.*

9   *To allow a comparison of patients between CEUC patients treated with azathioprine and those not so treated, rather than comparing with the general population.*

10 *For the primary study, the register had (apparently) only been kept for patients with inflammatory bowel disease who had been treated with azathioprine, so a similar control group simply was not available.*

11 *'Person-years at risk' is the cumulative total of years of observation for all the members of a group. Thus if a group of 200 patients at risk of cancer is followed up for a mean duration of 12 years, a total of 2400 person-years at risk have been observed.*

12 *The purpose of 'testing for significance' is to decide whether or not chance alone could be a reasonable explanation for any difference found between the groups. This should be contrasted with the idea of clinical importance (see Box 5.2).*

13 *Crohn's disease (in 450 of the 755 patients).*

14 *First, assume that the mean and median are similar (this may not always be so). We are told that 755 patients had a mean follow-up (from starting azathioprine) of 9.0 years. This yields $755 \times 9 = 6795$ person-years, close to the quoted figure of 6975 person-years.*

15 *17 (2%) of 755 patients lack information on final outcome: 11 emigrated and 6 others were lost sight of. 98% complete follow-up is very good.*

16 *The expected number of deaths (or cancer cases) is that which would occur if the group of patients experienced the same age/sex/time-specific mortality (or cancer incidence) as the general population. To calculate the expected number for each age/sex/calendar period, apply the appropriate national mortality rate to the number of patients concerned (see patients and methods section).*

17 *If the population of patients from which the sample is drawn and the general (national) population really had identical mortality experience and we repeatedly drew random samples of size 755 from the population, 19 times out of 20 the 95% confidence interval calculated for the sample drawn would include the true value. Since for our particular example zero is not included within the range, 'no difference' is a reasonable true population value, implying no statistically significant difference at the 5% level. (See also Box 5.1.)*

18   *About once in 20 000 repetitions of the study. This is calculated from the p value of 0.0001 given for rectal cancer in Table 2. Since the footnote indicates two-sided testing was used, the probability of getting seven or more cases of rectal cancer was 0.00005. You would therefore expect this result, which did in fact occur, only once in 20 000 repetitions. (Consult a statistical textbook for an explanation of two-sided testing.)*

19   *No: it is unreasonable to assume that the investigators have conducted the kind of study that happens only once in 10 000 times.*

20   *Colon, rectum, anal canal: all bowel-related sites.*

21   *We can see that patients with inflammatory bowel disease treated with azathioprine have an increased risk of developing bowel-related cancers – but we do not know whether this is as a result of the azathioprine or the inflammatory bowel disease itself, since both factors distinguish these patients from the general population.*

22   *Possibly, but we cannot be sure. As indicated in the last question, it may be the disease itself, not the treatment, which causes the excess risk.*

23   *Treatment for over 5 years.*

24   *No: the finding is consistent in all groups.*

25   *There is a consistent increase (double?) beyond 5 years of treatment for all cancers and for colorectal cancers specifically, whether Crohn's disease or ulcerative colitis is considered, but the authors do not mention these trends.*

      This adds some strength to the belief that azathioprine rather than (or as well as) inflammatory bowel disease is the cause of the increased risk. However, no specific test of statistical significance for this trend has been applied, simply tests of observed versus expected comparisons within one treatment period at a time. Of course, long periods of treatment with azathioprine probably also imply a long duration of inflammatory bowel disease, so this finding does not help us to disentangle the effects of the two exposures.

26   *0.91 expected among 282 patients (see Results text) with ulcerative colitis.*

27   *A = 8; B = 0.26; C = 6.19; D = 30.8; E = 1.3.*

28   *Row C, if we are interested in the risks of azathioprine in particular, rather than the risks of azathioprine and IBD together, since this allows us to isolate the **additional** risk posed by the treatment alone.*

29   *Yes, by comparison with the results in the secondary study. This would imply that the effects of azathioprine might not be as great as we might have thought.*

30   *'No significant difference' in the frequency of colorectal cancer between azathioprine-treated and other patients with 'extensive ulcerative colitis'. The authors do not provide confidence limits for this difference to enable us to judge whether the study was sufficiently large.*

31　*Once in 200 000 repetitions of the study under identical conditions (because p = 0.00001). See answer to question 18.*

32　*No, although question 25 above elicits some weak support from Table 3 for a dose–response effect, supporting at least a contributory effect by azathioprine. The confounding effect of duration of the disease itself has not been examined however.*

33　*A more cautious statement might read: 'The main study indicated that inflammatory bowel disease patients treated with azathioprine for 5 years or more may be at increased risk of cancer, especially colorectal cancer, but the smaller study of colorectal cancer risk in chronic extensive ulcerative colitis did not confirm any increase in risk.'*

34　*No, because risks associated with azathioprine treatment per se have been confounded with risks associated with inflamatory bowel disease in the main study, and while the secondary study did not show an increased risk due to azathioprine, the numbers of patients in that study may have been too small to show an effect, even if there was one.*

Checklist score: Our score was 56%

Our comment: The confounding of the effect of azathioprine and of inflammatory bowel disease on the incidence of neoplasia was an inherent weakness in this paper but it is doubtful whether the authors recognized it even at the analysis stage, let alone at the design stage.

EXERCISE 6

Introductory question:

a　*Patient specification: Full-term woman in labour with normal presentation of the fetus.*

b　*Intervention/exposure: Episiotomy.*

c　*Outcome of interest: Severe perineal tear.*

d　*Question using a, b, c: Does an episiotomy given to a woman in full-term labour with normal presentation of the fetus reduce the incidence of severe perineal tear?*

1　*Does the incidence of severe perineal trauma in vaginal deliveries differ where there is a policy of routinely administered episiotomy as opposed to a selective policy?*

2　*This paper uses the term 'trauma' rather than 'tear', and looks as though it will include a wider range of subjects. Only women who undergo caesarean deliveries will be excluded.*

3

a　*Admitted to one of eight hospitals with 'routine' policy.*

b　*August 1990–July 1992.*

c　*Informed consent.*

d　*Uncomplicated labour.*

e   *Nulliparous/primiparous gestation (first or second pregnancy).*

f   *Single fetus in cephalic presentation (i.e. head first).*

g   *No history of caesarean delivery or severe perineal tears.*

4   *Yes: they are equivalent to 'normal delivery'.*

5

a   *Selective episiotomy: try to avoid an episiotomy if possible and only do it for fetal indications or if severe perineal trauma was judged to be imminent.*

b   *Routine episiotomy: do an episiotomy according to the hospital's policy prior to the trial.*

6   *Yes: stratified by centre and parity, randomized blocks of 100. This is an unusually large block size (see Box 6.2) and may therefore not be effective in ensuring that within each stratum close to half the women are allocated to routine episiotomy and half to selective episiotomy.*

7   *By opening the next serially numbered envelope.*

8   *To ensure that the decision on whether or not a woman is admitted to the trial, or the order in which she is entered, occurs **before** medical staff identify which treatment the woman will receive if admitted now. Otherwise clinicians may consciously or unconsciously try to influence the treatment certain women receive, leading to the possibility of bias. Any contraindications to one treatment policy or the other should be exclusion criteria from the trial as a whole. (See Box 1.1 on blinding.)*

9   *Severe perineal trauma: defined as extension through the anal sphincter and/or the anal or rectal mucosa (third degree and fourth degree lacerations).*

10 *The investigators wanted to be able to detect a 50% increase in the real incidence of severe perineal trauma from 4% in routine episiotomy to 6% in selective episiotomy. Such differences are equivalent to a relative risk (RR) of 1.5 or to an attributable risk (AR) of 2%, or to one woman in 50 on the selective policy developing a tear 'due to' this policy.*

11

a   *'True' refers to the **theoretical** population of all such women from which the women **actually** admitted to the trial are assumed to be a random sample.*

b   *80%: this is the definition of 'statistical power'.*

12 *The categorical variables are oxytocin use, operative delivery, high birth weight (>3800 g) and previous episiotomy. The operative delivery proportion was a little higher in the routine group but for both groups this could be described as 'about 2%'. The other variables were very similar between the treatment groups.*

13   *The continuous variables are birth weight, cephalic perimeter and previous birth weight. These were very similar between the two groups, both in mean and standard deviation. The answers to this and the previous question suggest successful randomization.*

Statistical tests of significance (chi square test for categorical variables, t test or a non-parametric equivalent for continuous data) may be used to detect 'differences'. Absence of statistically significant differences may sometimes result from sample sizes which are too small rather than from the absence of any 'real' differences in the populations from which the samples come. For this reason a 'lower' level of statistical significance (e.g. 0.1 rather than 0.05) may be used to indicate those variables which it may be worth taking account of as 'confounders' or 'covariates' in the statistical analysis.

14   *These variables may plausibly be associated with a tear. We are not aware of others that should have been included, on the face of it, but specialists in the field may disagree.*

15

a   *Yes. The relative risk (selective vs routine) of SPT is the ratio of the risk of SPT in the selective sample to the risk of SPT in the routine sample.*

In the selective group: $15/1308 = 1.147\%$

In the routine group: $19/1298 = 1.463\%$

Hence: $RR = 1.147/1.463 = 0.78$

b   *Yes. The attributable risk in the selective sample compared to that in the routine sample is the **difference** in risk between them.*

$AR = 1.147\% - 1.463\%$

$= -0.32\%$ (to two decimal places)

(The negative sign indicates that, contrary to expectation, the risk is lower in the selective sample than in the routine one.)

c   *A number of explanations are possible. First, perhaps the risk of SPT had been exaggerated by supporters of episiotomy. Second, the estimate may have been based on historical data, and obstetric practice has improved. Third, the obstetricians/midwives in this study may have taken more care than usual, knowing they are under observation (this is termed the Hawthorne effect).*

16

a   *All of them, since all the 95% CIs include 1.*

b   *All of them, since all the 95% CIs include 0.*

c   *Yes, because the upper 95% confidence limit is only $+0.6\%$.*

d   *It has not been confirmed (this would require the lower 95% limit to exceed 1.5) but it has not been ruled out as it is a feasible real value, being contained within the 95% CI.*

17

    a   *At delivery: anterior perineal trauma and posterior perineal surgical repair.*

    b   *At discharge: perineal pain.*

    c   *At seventh day post-partum: healing complications and dehiscence.*

    Of these, only anterior perineal trauma has a RR (selective compared to routine) significantly (at the 5% level) higher than 1, indicating an advantage, here only, for routine episiotomy. However, note that the methods section does not indicate how many secondary outcomes were examined. We would expect 1 in 20 of such outcomes to show a statistically significant difference at the 5% level by chance alone.

18   *Reading from top to bottom of Table 3, the ARs (for the significant variables only, listed in the answer above) are:*

    +11.1%, −25.1%, −11.7%, −9.2%, −5.0%.

    Whereas the selective episiotomy has an attributable risk of 11% for anterior perineal trauma, this is offset by the −12% AR for perineal pain. However, the largest attributable risk (−25%) is for posterior perineal surgical repair for which the selective episiotomy therefore apparently has a great advantage. One quarter of women on a routine episiotomy would apparently be spared posterior perineal surgical repair if managed selectively instead. Clinical judgement is needed to weigh up these advantages and disadvantages. (See discussion.)

19   *A = Not given in the paper; B = Not given in the paper; C = 2606; D = 1308; E = 1298; F = 1.2%; G = 0; H = 1.5%; I = 0.*

20   *Yes: apart from the 'materials and methods' section saying so, the flow chart confirms that results of the primary outcome measure are compared between the two groups of patients as they appeared immediately after randomization.*

21   *Only 30% of the selective group had an episiotomy, compared to 83% of the routine group.*

22   *'1.2%–0.6%' should read '−1.2% to 0.6%'.*

23   *Not really: our consideration of attributable risk led us to focus on the advantage of selective episiotomy in posterior perineal surgical repairs (AR = −25%), whereas the authors have emphasized the same variable, quoting the 28% reduction in relative risk. They then mention, correctly, only the other statistically significant changes in Table 3.*

24

a   *100 patients treated by selective rather than routine episiotomy have been estimated (our most reliable estimate) to prevent 0.317 cases of SPT. In other words, about 315 cases (100/0.317) need to be treated to prevent one case: NNT = 315.*

b   *1.2% is the highest (negative end) 95% confidence limit given. This would correspond to NNT = 100/1.2 = 83, the lowest reasonable NNT if 'selective' better than 'routine'.*

c   *0.6% is the highest (positive end) 95% confidence limit given. This would correspond to NNT = 100/0.6 = 167, the lowest reasonable NNT if 'routine' better than 'selective'.*

25   *Yes.*

26   *Fetal outcome measures were not mentioned in the methods section. The only direct measure of fetal outcome is the 1-minute Apgar score (on a 0–10 scale) which did not change significantly (Table 3).*

27   *Yes: use episiotomy selectively.*

Checklist score: Our score was 86%

Our comment: The expected (by the authors) benefit of routine episiotomy was not confirmed in this trial. What was particularly surprising was that the incidence of severe perineal tear, anticipated at 4–6%, was under 2% in both treatment groups. Statistical power calculations therefore underestimated the number of patients needed to detect an increase of 50% in incidence. A bigger study was really needed.

EXERCISE 7

1   *What variables predict the men with disseminated prostate cancer who are likely to die of their disease?*

2   *A representative sample of newly diagnosed patients with disseminated disease (subjects), an assessment of potentially useful variables (measureent), and a measure of survival time/ proportion alive by a given length of follow-up (outcome).*

3   *Because it is important to classify patients into (high/low) risk groups so as to select appropriate treatments. We might also want to classify patients in this way for information (for example to help counsel patients or relatives), or as a basis for stratification in future evaluations of treatment or observational studies of new prognostic factors.*

4   *September 1984 to January 1988.*

5   *Two clinical trials – one of Zoladex and one of orchiectomy. Note that the patients did not come from a trial of Zoladex vs orchiectomy.*

6   *191.*

7   *Because 16 had advanced **local** disease (i.e. invading structures such as rectum or bladder). Such patients are qualitatively different – their disease might be treatable by local (if radical) surgery for example, and their prognosis might be determined more by effects on the kidneys as opposed to the general 'tumour burden' of metastatic disease.*

8   *A = ? (insufficient data in text); B = 75; C = ?; D = ?; E = 116; F = ? (but C + F = 16); G = 175.*

9

a   *We do not know, as from this paper we cannot tell how selective the eligibility criteria for the original clinical trials were, nor the proportion of patients agreeing to take part. This matters because the representativeness of the patients will reflect the clinical usefulness of the prognostic variables identified by the authors.*

b   *At first sight yes (newly diagnosed metastatic disease) but metastatic disease can be diagnosed while still asymptomatic – if regular checks are made such as X-ray or biochemical tests; it is not specified here whether regular checks like this were done or whether patients were just expected to turn up when they developed symptoms. The studies referred to by the authors would need to be reviewed for this information.*

10   *About 5 years.*

11

a   *Patient – age, performance status*

Tumour – tumour grade, extent (area of bone involvement)
Treatment – Zoladex, orchiectomy (pooled in this instance as they gave similar hormone deprivation)

b   *Age is a continuous variable, performance status is ordinal, tumour grade is ordinal, extent is continuous (but constrained in the range 0,100%), treatment is category.*

12   *More recent work has looked at the presence of oncogene markers such as p53 or c-myc as possible predictors of survival. Another possibility is the rate of change of PSA levels (analogous to HCG) – but it seems they included the potentially important variables known at the time.*

13   *No. The authors state that '...survival was considered with respect only to deaths related to cancer...'.*

14   *Time to tumour progression and time to death from prostate cancer.*

15   *The first outcome has the same limitations as the original diagnosis of metastatic disease – although a definition is given we lack protocol details; the second is objective in the fact of death, but criteria for ascribing the cause to prostate cancer (and evidence of their reproducibility) are lacking.*

Whether they are free from bias depends principally on whether the diagnosis of progression/death from prostate cancer was made by someone blind to the values of each patient's prognostic factors.

16   *Kaplan–Meier based survival plots (see Box 7.1) and the log-rank test and by Cox regression for significance tests and estimation of the prognostic index (see Boxes 7.2 and 7.3).*

17

a   *The authors do not say.*

b   *82, with 68 dying of prostate cancer.*

18

a   *$83/(83 + 90) = 48\%$. Note that two patients did not have a haemoglobin done at all.*

b   *Those with a haemoglobin level of less than 8.5, because their 2-year survival was 48% but those aged 60–70 years had a 2-year survival of 61%.*

c   *The P value for testosterone is very small, and indicates the 'unlikeliness' of finding the observed association between testosterone and survival if in fact testosterone was really unrelated to survival. The caveat here is that this is not a randomized controlled trial, so that this observation may actually represent the biasing effect of some other, unmeasured factor.*

19   *Log relative risk = (beta coefficient) · (value of variable). Here haemoglobin is recoded to two values: >8.5 (coded as 0) and <8.5 (coded as 1), and the beta coefficient is 0.5. So log relative risk $= 0.5 \cdot 1 = 0.5$, and relative risk $= exp(0.5) = 1.65$.*

20   *Now there are three variables. Haemoglobin is coded by one dummy variable as above. PS is coded as two dummy variables, each with its own beta coefficient: both are coded as 0 if PS = 100%. If PS is 60–90% the first dummy is coded as 1, the second as 0. If PS is <60% the first dummy is coded as 0 and the second as 1. Hence the total log relative risk $= 0.5 \cdot 1 + 0.85 \cdot 0 + 0.95 \cdot 1$, so relative risk $= exp(0.5 + 0.95) = 4.26$.*

21   *The univariate analysis looks at the effect of one variable (e.g. grade) on survival; the 'multivariate' one – Cox regression – allows the joint effect of several variables to be assessed simultaneously, in effect adjusting for possible correlations that may exist between the variables.*

22   *A univariate analysis is a useful 'screen' and is in effect normally done on the first step of a 'stepwise' regression; it is the multivariate one that is really useful though, as it shows the effect of each variable having allowed for the effects of the others (often referred to as the 'independent' effect of the variable).*

23

a   *Performance status and alkaline phosphatase.*

b   *P < 0.1 which would increase the risk of thinking a variable was related to outcome, when in reality it is not.*

24

a   *They can be thought of as indicating the 'smear of uncertainty' surrounding an estimated value, because another sample would not be expected to give exactly the same answer; or as a range of 'plausible' alternatives.*

b   *We do not know as they were not given, nor were the standard errors.*

25   *By plotting a survival curve for each group, or tabulating some summary figure such as median survival time. Better still, a separate sample of patients could be classified by these prognostic groups and the survival plots displayed. This is an example of cross-validation. Usually the difference between the prognostic categories turns out to be not as great on a new set of patients as when applied to the original data.*

26

a   *About 40%.*

b   *The assumption concerns the proportion of deaths in men with metastatic prostate cancer that are due to the disease. Figure 1 refers to prostate cancer-**specific** survival. You could either assume all such men die of the cancer, or you could take the figure of 68/82, since from the results section we know that 82 men died, 68 of them from prostate cancer.*

This assumes that this proportion of cancer-specific deaths is the same in all prognostic groups – which implies an overall survival that is definitely worse.

c   *You cannot tell until at least 50% have died (think: what is the definition of median survival?) and this was not the case here. The study ended before half of the men in this group had died.*

27   *The **good** group is men with (a) low Alk P, plus (b) unimpaired PS/slightly impaired PS, plus (c) no anaemia.*

*The **bad** group is men with (a) high Alk P, plus (b) impaired PS/slightly impaired PS, plus (c) anaemia.*

*The **intermediate** group is anyone not in the good or bad group.*

By 3 years all the bad group, half the moderate group and a third of the good group will have died of prostate cancer.

28

a   *They do not mention any!*

b

i   *The representativeness of the patients – this is not really established. Ideally we would have a breakdown by age, and we would need information on the proportions who were ineligible for the original trials.*

ii   *The total numbers assessed for the various prognostic factors are not all 175 so the analyses cannot be based on all the patients. The discrepancy is not mentioned. Beware this 'ice-erg' of numbers that do not add up. This may be just typographical error or it could have more profound implications. For example, testosterone was only measured on 59 subjects so could not have been included in a multivariate analysis on more than these subjects.*

iii Statistics: the significance level for the multivariate analysis is unusually high yet it was not discussed. Also confidence limits for the regression coefficients were not given, so we have no idea how precise these were. Tests for trend in survival do not seem to have been applied (e.g. for age, T status, PS and other ordered scales), which would have been more powerful.

iv Methodology: the prognostic factors were categorized to define the prognostic groups, rather than define these on the basis of percentiles of the prognostic index, and no cross-validation of the index was made. Cross-validation would have involved, for example, trying out the prognostic groupings on a new sample of patients to see how well it performed; the same approach could have been used to see if the same prognostic variables were selected. Neither was there any description of the goodness of fit of their index, which would indicate the extent to which a search for new prognostic variables could be useful.

29 (Readers to provide)

30

a Within the limitations described above, yes.

b No.

31 How applicable is the index of prognosis to other prostate cancer patients; will it be affected by new treatments; what about longer term prognosis for the 'good' group?

32 Yes, but with caution as the uncertainty is not quantified.

Checklist score: Our score was 69%

Our comment: A study that proved less useful than appeared at first sight, because of flaws in the statistical analysis (not all variables measured on each subject, no confidence limits on regression coefficients, and no validation). Moreover the survival was with respect only to death from prostate cancer and so could mislead the unwary.

EXERCISE 8

1 To determine which clinical features can be used to distinguish between a high or low risk of thromboembolism in placebo-treated patients with non-rheumatic atrial fibrillation.

2 Placebo-treated patients with non-rheumatic atrial fibrillation (AF) (type of patient), measurements of likely prognostic variables (measurements), follow-up to measure occurrence of thrombo-embolism (outcome).

3 Because trials of anticoagulants used careful patient selection and strict protocols to reduce the risk of untoward bleeding; for routine clinical practice it would help maximize the benefit/risk ratio if patients with a high risk of embolism could be identified in the first place.

4 1987–1989.

5 They were the placebo groups from a multicentre trial (in '15 clinical centres') of warfarin vs aspirin vs placebo.

6   *568*

7

    A = ?

    B = 1330

    C = 568

8

a   *Up to a point, yes. They were recruited from outpatient and inpatient departments of a variety of hospital types, but we do not know in what proportions. The references cited might take us further.*

b   *It is not stated.*

9

a   *The idea is to assess the risk of stroke or other embolism in patients originally given no anticoagulant irrespective of any subsequent changes to their treatment.*

b   *This will give an estimate of the net risks including any modification to the risk induced by normal clinical practice.*

10   *None, the authors report 'complete follow-up of all placebo assigned groups'.*

11   *No. The authors state that 'enlisted patients were those without... prosthetic valves'.*

12   *By 3-monthly follow-up with review of the medical notes by a committee that was unaware of the patients' treatment (for the significance of this method, refer to Box 1.1).*

13   *The outcomes are potentially objective, although criteria for ischaemic stroke are not given (but might be available in other reports of the trial). The method of assessment means they should also be free from bias.*

14   *Since there were 46 primary thromboembolic events, between 2 and 4 (46/20 to 46/10).*

15   *By Poisson regression (essentially a person-years method) for actual risks, and by Cox regression to evaluate the relative risks, plus an 'exact' method. For more information on these methods, see Boxes 7.3 and 8.2.*

16

a   *Patient: age, sex.*

    Disease: duration of AF, intermittent AF.

    Treatments: diuretics, pacemaker.

b   *Age is continuous (but displayed as ordinal), and the others are all presented as categories though are potentially at least ordinal.*

c   *Information is lost when continuous data such as height are reduced to a dichotomy (such as >6 ft vs ≤6 ft). If it has to be done an optimum cut-point can be defined in the sense of one that preserves as much of the original variance as possible.*

17   *Apparently not, the* a priori *and literature-derived factors should have sufficed, although it is not clear why the additional clinical variables were introduced. Factors should be chosen if they are likely to affect outcome; in this sense even treatment can be regarded as a prognostic factor, and it is arguable that prognostic factors should always be evaluated taking into account treatment received.*

18

a   *Patients with recent congestive heart failure (17.7% per year).*

b   *The 76+ age group (ratio of upper 95% confidence limit (UCL) to lower 95% confidence limit (LCL) = 5.1).*

19

a   *A never decreasing upward trend.*

b   *The magnitudes of the relative risks have all fallen, giving a truer picture of their **independent** effects (i.e. the part not accounted for by the other variables). The precision (as shown by UCL/LCL ratio) of the relative risks of hypertension and recent heart failure has fallen, whereas that associated with previous thromboembolism has risen.*

20   *It has probably been entered as a continuous variable, in 10-year units (the footnote says age was entered by decade).*

21

a   *As high risk.*

b   *As low risk.*

c   *By constructing a life-table (survival) plot (see Box 7.1).*

22

a   *(40 years (20–78) if no risk factors present.)*

     14 years (9–21) if one risk factor present.

     6 years (3–10) if two or three risk factors present.

b   *Yes, 4 years is well outside the 95% confidence interval for people with no risk factors present. The same applies for people with one risk factor present.*

     For people with two or three risk factors it would not be unusual, because the 95% confidence interval includes 4 years.

23   *In otherwise low risk patients.*

24

a   *The secondary analyses, i.e. ones not specified as necessary to test the hypothesis at the beginning of the study, but more exploratory in nature. Differing definitions of variables between studies, which can also cause problems of comparability.*

b

i   *As above, but with the addition that no reasons were given for the additional clinical variables. The P values for the secondary analyses, and for the additional clinical variables, need to be regarded with suspicion, as being indicative and without apparent correction for multiple significance testing. On the other hand the main indicators were stable.*

ii   *Perhaps more important is that no validation was given (it could be internal, on a leave-one-out basis, or on a new data set). See Box 8.1 for more information.*

25   *We will not do this for you, but similar abstracts are created for publication in the* ACP Journal Club *and* Evidence Based Medicine *(see Appendix II).*

26   *Yes.*

27   *There is still the matter of the kinds of patient who were ineligible for the original trial.*

28

a   *Yes.*

b   *Only in part. We can estimate the risk of a stroke in this man. He has one risk factor, implying a stroke in 9–21 years, but we do not know what the risk of side-effects would be if he was treated. The introduction quotes a highest risk of 2.5% per year for a 'serious bleeding complication'. This is not enough – you should have done the MEDLINE search and looked at the SPAF study!*

Checklist score: Our score was 78%

Our comment: A nice paper that looks pretty useful. The main questions were how objective the outcome measure (stroke) is (could minor lesions have been missed by some centres?) and a risk of overfitting because the number of events was only 46, suggesting that it would be unwise to look for more than three or four variables. The authors could have set our minds at rest by a cross-validation exercise.

EXERCISE 9

1   *Do patients with strokes (the population) managed in specialist stroke units (the intervention) have improved survival (the outcome), as compared with conventional treatment?*

2   *Time to full recovery*

    Time to discharge from hospital

    Functional outcome (i.e. ability to perform certain everyday tasks)

    Each of these outcomes, as well as survival, would be of interest to you as a policymaker.

3   *They might have carried out a new piece of primary research – probably a randomized trial of stroke units versus conventional management. Instead, they have chosen to look at previously reported research, in the hope of combining the results in some way to reach a firm conclusion. If sufficient evidence already exists in research already done, this may be a very much quicker and cheaper way to answer the question than starting a new study from scratch.*

Research based on already collected data or conclusions from previous studies is known as secondary research.

4 *They searched citations listed in Index Medicus, MEDLINE, conference abstracts, bibliographies, textbooks and reviews. They also spoke to colleagues and other researchers in the area.*

5 *The stated inclusion criteria are:*

randomized controlled trial

subjects of the trial are patients with acute stroke

the control group is managed in general medicine/neurology wards

the intervention group is managed in a 'stroke unit' which includes a multidisciplinary team of specialists.

Although they do not say so explicitly, all the studies must also record mortality as an outcome.

6 *It is debatable whether the definition of a stroke unit is sufficiently precise. As the authors state, the criterion used could apply to a 'physical' stroke unit, such as a dedicated ward for patients with stroke, as well as a 'virtual' stroke unit, such as a stroke team which visits patients being cared for on conventional medical wards. The only thing all forms of 'stroke unit' care must have in common in their definition is a multidisciplinary team. One might also question what defines such a team, and whether it can be clearly distinguished from the loosely affiliated team of health professionals who care for stroke patients in conventional settings.*

On the other hand, more tightly drawn criteria may have resulted in only one or two studies being eligible for the review.

7 *We are unable to make a clear judgement about this, since we are not given any information on the search terms used for the MEDLINE search. A poor search strategy on MEDLINE might easily miss a number of important trials. In addition, other databases could have been searched, although it is likely that most important studies will have been published in journals indexed by MEDLINE.*

8 *Unpublished trials may remain unpublished for a number of reasons. One reason may be that they do not show any benefit from the intervention of interest ('negative trials'), and so are judged to be less interesting than trials that do show a benefit. Another reason may be that a trial is judged un-publishable because it is too small to have a good chance of showing statistical significance, even if real, clinically important differences exist.*

If such evidence is excluded from consideration in a systematic review, there may be a bias towards including studies with positive results – 'publication bias'.

9 *Two of the researchers 'independently assessed reports to confirm eligibility criteria and results', but it is not clear whether this assessment extended to a judgement of the overall quality of each study.*

10   *An intention to treat analysis compares outcomes for individuals according to the treatment status to which they were **originally allocated**, rather than according to the treatment which they may actually have **received**. A fuller discussion of this topic can be found in Box 9.3.*

This is entirely appropriate in a pragmatic study which aims to discover whether there are benefits to a particular mode of service organization in the real world.

11   *Randomization: eight trials used a formal randomization, and two did not.*

Intervention: five trials evaluated a distinct stroke ward/team, and five evaluated an extension to usual rehabilitation. We are also given information about some of the differences in extent and timing of therapies which resulted.

Subjects: all trials had a common definition of stroke, but not of inclusion/exclusion criteria.

Outcome: mortality data were obtained for all trials, though were not in the original publication in two cases.

12   *There are a number of possibilities. One approach would be simply to select whichever trial(s) you feel are the 'best', and ignore the others. Another would be to see whether the majority of the trials support one particular conclusion.*

However, these methods would not help if all of the trials are inconclusive, or if some trials reach one conclusion and apparently equally good trials reach the opposite conclusion. What we really need is a technique to combine the results from all of the trials, as if a new trial were being performed which included all of the patients for whom we already have data.

*Such a quantitative method of combining results is termed **meta-analysis**. Details of the various methods of meta-analysis are beyond the scope of this book. Only the broad principles are explained here.*

13   *The odds ratio tells us the odds of death in the intervention group compared to that in the controls. An odds ratio of less than 1 implies some benefit from stroke units, whereas an odds ratio greater than 1 implies that they are harmful. The 95% CI tells us the range of values within which the actual odds ratio may plausibly lie.*

To be sure of benefit, we want the upper 95% confidence limit to be less than 1. If the range includes values greater than 1, then it would be plausible that stroke units have no effect, or even harm patients.

14

a   *Only one of the trials (Indredavik) has resulted in an odds ratio with a confidence interval which is wholly less than 1. In all the other trials, the CI extends to values greater than 1, indicating uncertainty over benefit. We are therefore faced with a single positive trial and nine inconclusive trials, which might make us doubtful that definite benefit existed.*

    b   *For mortality at 1 year, seven of the trials suggest some benefit, but none are conclusive since the CI for each of them extends above 1. We could not reach a conclusion about the effects of stroke unit care on 1-year mortality from any of these trials taken individually.*

15   *The text and figures do match. There is a 28% reduction in the odds of death within 17 weeks, and a 21% reduction in the odds of death within 12 months. Though not calculated explicitly here, the number needed to be treated (NNT) to save one life is about 15.*

16   *They calculate what the combined odds ratio would be after the inclusion of (imaginary) results from those trials, assuming that the trials were to show no benefit.*

    Similarly, they consider the possible impact of publication bias by calculating how many patients would be required in neutral trials to alter the conclusions of the meta-analysis. This method has been criticized, however, for the assumption that un-published studies would be neutral.

17   *The general strategy the authors adopt is to exclude trials or results about which they have doubts, and then recalculate a combined odds ratio from the remaining data. In this way they can test whether the conclusions are altered by imposing a higher level of methodological rigour.*

    For example, they exclude the two trials with informal random-ization to see whether this affects the conclusion. In another trial in which randomization has resulted in differences between the groups, they exclude all patients with reduced conscious level and reanalyse the remaining patients.

18   *The authors address this point. They argue that no trial showed poorer functional status, and nine showed some improvement in functional status, in patients managed in stroke units compared to those managed conventionally. However, we do not know whether the individual studies were powerful enough to detect clinically relevant changes in morbidity outcomes.*

19   *The authors seem to be arguing as follows: because most of the trials indicated that treatment in a stroke unit confers a small reduction in the odds of death, and the size of this reduction was similar across the trials, we can conclude that the component of the care which actually produces this effect must be the same in each of the stroke units.*

    We would argue that this conclusion does not logically follow. Because we are uncertain about what exactly is entailed by stroke unit care in each of the trials, it is entirely possible that trial A might produce a 20% fall in mortality due to some therapy A, while in trial B a similar fall is produced by some therapy B. It would also be conceivable that trial C, in which intervention patients received both therapies A and B, would achieve mortality benefits much greater than 20%. This is a variant of the 'ecological fallacy'.

20   *That care of patients in stroke units is associated with sustained improvements in survival.*

21   *Yes. The results of the meta-analysis are unambiguous. The whole confidence interval for each overall odds ratio is less than 1. Nonetheless, some ambiguity remains over the nature of the intervention which has been shown to have this beneficial effect.*

22   *Are local stroke patients similar (in age, diagnosis, stroke severity) to those included in the trials?*

      Is the outcome (mortality) relevant and the size of the effect (over 20% reduction in odds ratio) important?

      Is the local intervention likely to be similar to those evaluated in these trials?

23   *Yes, the paper has helped: you are now able to explain to your colleagues that although some studies were inconclusive or contradictory, nonetheless when all the evidence is considered together there appears to be a benefit (in terms of survival) to stroke unit care.*

      This knowledge may mean that the planning team will now want to recommend the establishment of such a service locally. However, many uncertainties still remain over how this should best be done. It is clear that a multidisciplinary team is required, but what else? Is a separate ward needed? Should the service treat stroke patients of any age? Is it better to concentrate on patients with mild stroke or those with severe stroke? And how much would a new service like this cost?

      *Although this paper has helped you, you now face many more questions about how a new service should be established. In a useful follow up to this paper, these issues are discussed in detail (Dennis M, Langhorne P. So stroke units save lives: where do we go from here? Br Med J 1994; **309:** 1273–1277).*

      Checklist score: Our score was 83%

APPENDIX 1 Checklists for critical appraisal

Many checklists have been devised for evaluating the quality of published articles in the medical literature. Six adaptations have been developed for use with the six distinct types of exercise in this book:

1 Clinical agreement.

2 Diagnosis/screening.

3 Causation/harm.

4 Therapy.

5 Prognosis.

6 Overview.

We have drawn primarily on the 'users' guides' to the medical literature shown in the reference list, adapting as follows:

- We listed all the questions in the six relevant users' guides, and recognized that some questions phrased as single sentences were complex and could be broken into components.

- We wanted to derive a crude overall score to assess the quality and usefulness of the article and, as a starting point have worded all the questions so that 'yes' means 'good' and scores 2, while 'No' means 'poor' and scores 0. Some questions are 'not applicable' and should effectively be ignored, not counted as 0. Questions are sometimes difficult or unclear and the answer to such a question should score 1.

- Six prototype checklists along these lines were devised by one of us (PBS), corresponding to each of the types of article critically appraised in this book.

- Two of the authors (RAD, PBS) and another colleague (MB) tried out all checklists except that on overview, on our own, then with 230 medical students working in groups of six, and subsequently in reaching consensus among the three of us.

- We further adapted the checklist to remove ambiguities, though doubtless some remain. These checklists are attached and may be photocopied as needed.

We plan further work on inter- and intra-rater agreement.

References

1. CLINICAL AGREEMENT

   Clinical disagreement: I. How often it occurs and why. *CMA J* 1980; **123:** 499–504

   Clinical disagreement: II. How to avoid it and how to learn from one's mistakes. *CMA J* 1980; **123:** 613–617

2. DIAGNOSIS/SCREENING

   Jaeschke R, Guyatt G, and Sackett DL. Users' guides to the medical literature: III. How to use an article about a diagnostic test (part A). Are the results of the study valid? *JAMA* 1994; **271:** 389–391

   Jaeschke R, Guyatt GH, and Sackett DL. Users' guides to the medical literature: III. How to use an article about a diagnostic test (part B). What are the results and will they help me in caring for my patients? *JAMA* 1994; **271:** 703–707

3. CAUSATION/HARM

   Levine M, Walter S, Lee H, Haines T, Holbrook A, and Moyer V. Users' guides to the medical literature: IV. How to use an article about harm. *JAMA* 1994; **271:** 1615–1619

4. THERAPY

   Guyatt GH, Sackett DL, and Cook DJ. Users' guides to the medical literature: II. How to use an article about therapy or prevention (part A). Are the results of the study valid? *JAMA* 1993; **270:** 2598–2601

   Guyatt GH, Sackett DL, and Cook DJ. Users' guides to the medical literature: II. How to use an article about therapy or prevention (part B). What were the results and will they help me in caring for my patients? *JAMA* 1994; **271:** 59–63

5. PROGNOSIS

   Laupacis A, Wells G, Richardson S, and Tugwell P. Users' guides to the medical literature: V. How to use an article about prognosis. *JAMA* 1994; **272:** 234–237

6. OVERVIEW

   Oxman AD, Cook DJ, and Guyatt GH. Users' guides to the medical literature: VI. How to use an overview. *JAMA* 1994; **272:** 1367–1371

7. QUALITY OF CARE

   How to read clinical journals: VI. To learn about the quality of clinical care. *Can Med Assoc J* 1984; **130:** 377–381

8. ECONOMIC EVALUATION

   How to read clinical journals: VII. To understand an economic evaluation (part A). *Can Med Assoc J* 1984; **130:** 1428–1433

   How to read clinical journals: VII. To understand an economic evaluation (part B). *Can Med Assoc J* 1984; **130:** 1542–1549

9. CLINICAL DECISION ANALYSIS

   Scott Richardson W and Detsky AS. Users' guides to the medical literature: VII. How to use a Clinical Decision Analysis. A. Are the results of the study valid? *JAMA* 1995; **273:** 1292–1295

   Scott Richardson W and Detsky AS. Users' guides to the medical literature: VII. How to use a Clinical Decision Analysis. B. What are the results and will they help me in caring for my patients? *JAMA* 1995; **273:** 1610–1613

10. CLINICAL PRACTICE GUIDELINES

   Hayward RSA, Wilson MC, Tunis SR, Bass EB, and Guyatt G. Users' guides to the medical literature: VIII. How to use clinical practice guidelines. A. Are the recommendations valid? *JAMA* 1995; **274:** 570–574

11. GENERAL INTRODUCTION TO USERS' GUIDES

   Guyatt G, Rennie D and the Evidence Based Medicine Working Group. Why Users' Guides? EBM Working Paper Series #1. Only available on the Internet as:

   http://HIRU.MCMASTER.CA/ebm/0_users.htm

   Oxman AD, Sackett DL, and Guyatt GH. Users' guide to the medical literature: I. How to get started. *JAMA* 1993; **270:** 2093–2095. Also available on the Internet as: http://HIRU.MCMASTER.CA/ebm/userguid/1_intro.htm

RATING SCALE 1 FOR ARTICLE ON CLINICAL AGREEMENT

	Yes	Unclear/ possibly	No	Not applicable
			Ring the appropriate code	
RESULTS				
1 Is the aim clearly posed?	2	1	0	N/A
2 Is it clear why the study was needed?	2	1	0	N/A
VALIDITY				
Subjects				
3 Is where they came from specified?	2	1	0	N/A
4 Is how they were chosen specified?	2	1	0	N/A
5 Is why they were chosen specified?	2	1	0	N/A
Raters				
6 Is where they came from specified?	2	1	0	N/A
7 Is how they were chosen specified?	2	1	0	N/A
8 Is why they were chosen specified?	2	1	0	N/A
9 Were they 'blinded' to other information?	2	1	0	N/A
10 If 'No', is method of presenting this information given?	2	1	0	N/A
Conditions of study				
11 Were Routine ('Normal' conditions) used?	2	1	0	N/A
12 Were the same conditions maintained throughout?	2	1	0	N/A
13 Was special training needed?	2	1	0	N/A
14 If 'Yes', did those who needed it, get it?	2	1	0	N/A
Statistical analysis				
15 Were methods used appropriate?	2	1	0	N/A
16 Were 'special' methods justified by authors?	2	1	0	N/A
RESULTS				
Inter-observer agreement:				
17 Is reproducibility satisfactory?	2	1	0	N/A
18 Is the result adequately precise?	2	1	0	N/A
19 Was chance agreement allowed for?	2	1	0	N/A
Intra-observer agreement				
20 Is reproducibility satisfactory?	2	1	0	N/A
21 Is the result adequately precise?	2	1	0	N/A
22 Was chance agreement allowed for?	2	1	0	N/A
Accuracy (i.e. vs 'gold standard')				
23 Was the 'gold standard' appropriate?	2	1	0	N/A
24 Is the result adequately precise?	2	1	0	N/A
25 Was chance agreement allowed for?	2	1	0	N/A
UTILITY				
26 Will the results alter my practice?	2	1	0	N/A

TOTAL (add ringed scores above): _____ **(A)**

No. of questions which actually applied to this article (maximum = 26): _____ **(B)**

Maximum possible score (2 × B): _____ **(C)**

OVERALL RATING (A/C expressed as a percentage): _____ %

COMMENTS:

RATING SCALE 2 FOR ARTICLE ON DIAGNOSIS/SCREENING

	Yes	Unclear/ possibly	No	Not applicable
		Ring the appropriate code		

RESULTS

		Yes	Unclear/ possibly	No	Not applicable
1	Are likelihood ratios (or necessary data) given?	2	1	0	N/A
2	Is the 'best cutpoint' of clinical importance?	2	1	0	N/A
	(i.e. can the test usefully distinguish those with the disease from those without?)	2	1	0	N/A
3	Is the estimate of sensitivity/specificity (or likelihood ratio) sufficiently precise?	2	1	0	N/A

VALIDITY

Selection

		Yes	Unclear/ possibly	No	Not applicable
4	Was the phase of the disease well defined?	2	1	0	N/A
5	Were patients at a uniform point in this phase?	2	1	0	N/A
6	Was the origin of the population of potential subjects (study population) described?	2	1	0	N/A

Measurement

		Yes	Unclear/ possibly	No	Not applicable
7	Was assessment against the gold standard 'blind'	2	1	0	N/A
8	Was the 'gold standard' applied to all subjects independent of the test result?	2	1	0	N/A
9	Could I repeat the study using the methods as described?	2	1	0	N/A
10	Was the repeatability of the test assessed?	2	1	0	N/A

Statistical analysis

		Yes	Unclear/ possibly	No	Not applicable
11	Were additional factors that might modify the test result (e.g. age, sex, disease phase) allowed for?	2	1	0	N/A
12	Were appropriate methods used?	2	1	0	N/A
13	Were any 'unusual' methods explained or justified?	2	1	0	N/A
	(e.g. are methods easily found in a standard textbook – lots of references in MEDLINE? If so, it is probably not unusual)				

UTILITY

		Yes	Unclear/ possibly	No	Not applicable
14	For those who test positive do the results help me choose among alternative actions/treatments?	2	1	0	N/A
15	For those who test negative do the results help me reassure/counsel patients?	2	1	0	N/A

TOTAL (add ringed scores above): _____ **(A)**

No. of questions which actually applied to this article (maximum = 15): _____ **(B)**

Maximum possible score (2 × B): _____ **(C)**

OVERALL RATING (A/C expressed as a percentage): _____ %

COMMENTS:

RATING SCALE 3 FOR ARTICLE ON CAUSATION (OR HARM)

		Ring the appropriate code			
		Yes	Unclear/ possibly	No	Not applicable
RESULTS					
1	Is an estimate of association between exposure and outcome given?	2	1	0	N/A
2	Is it of clinical importance?	2	1	0	N/A
3	Is it sufficiently precise to be useful?	2	1	0	N/A
VALIDITY					
Selection					
4	Was the diagnosis of the disease well defined?	2	1	0	N/A
5	Was the source of the cases/cohort described?	2	1	0	N/A
6	Were efforts made to ensure complete ascertainment of cases?	2	1	0	N/A
Measurement					
7	Were all subjects accounted for?	2	1	0	N/A
8	Were losses to follow-up/refusals low (<10%)?	2	1	0	N/A
9	Were outcomes and/or exposures measured alike in all groups?	2	1	0	N/A
10	Was assessment of exposure objective?	2	1	0	N/A
Statistical analysis					
11	Were additional factors allowed for?	2	1	0	N/A
12	Were appropriate methods used?	2	1	0	N/A
13	Were any 'unusual' methods explained or justified?	2	1	0	N/A
14	Was a 'dose–response' gradient demonstrated?	2	1	0	N/A
15	Was the temporal relationship correct?	2	1	0	N/A
UTILITY					
16	Do the results help me choose treatments or avoid exposures?	2	1	0	N/A
17	Do the results help me reassure/counsel patients?	2	1	0	N/A

TOTAL (add ringed scores above): _____ **(A)**

No. of questions which actually applied to this article (maximum = 17): _____ **(B)**

Maximum possible score (2 × B): _____ **(C)**

OVERALL RATING (A/C expressed as a percentage): _____ %

COMMENTS:

RATING SCALE 4 FOR ARTICLE ON THERAPY

	Ring the appropriate code			
	Yes	Unclear/ possibly	No	Not applicable
RESULTS				
1 Is an estimate of the treatment effect given?	2	1	0	N/A
2 Is it of clinical importance?	2	1	0	N/A
3 Is the estimate of treatment effect sufficiently precise?	2	1	0	N/A
VALIDITY				
Selection				
4 Was the spectrum of patients well defined?	2	1	0	N/A
5 Was the diagnosis of the disease well defined?	2	1	0	N/A
6 If pragmatic, were suitably broad eligibility criteria used?	2	1	0	N/A
7 If explanatory, were eligibility criteria suitably narrow?	2	1	0	N/A
Measurement				
8 Was assignment to treatments stated to be random?	2	1	0	N/A
9 If yes, was the method of randomization explained?	2	1	0	N/A
10 Were all patients accounted for after randomization?	2	1	0	N/A
11 Were losses to follow-up low (<10%)?	2	1	0	N/A
12 Were the treatment groups similar in important factors at the start of the trial?	2	1	0	N/A
13 Were all patients otherwise treated alike?	2	1	0	N/A
14 Were patients, health care workers and investigators 'blind' to treatment?	2	1	0	N/A
15 Was assessment of outcome 'blind'?	2	1	0	N/A
16 Was the occurrence of side-effects explicitly looked for?	2	1	0	N/A
17 If yes, were estimates of their frequency/severity given?	2	1	0	N/A
Statistical analysis				
18 Was the main analysis on 'intention to treat'?	2	1	0	N/A
19 If no, was a sensitivity analysis performed?	2	1	0	N/A
20 Were additional clinically relevant factors allowed for?	2	1	0	N/A
21 Were appropriate statistical methods used?	2	1	0	N/A
22 Were any 'unusual' methods explained or justified?	2	1	0	N/A
23 If subgroup analyses were done, were they explicitly presented as such?	2	1	0	N/A
UTILITY				
24 Do the results help me choose treatments?	2	1	0	N/A

TOTAL (add ringed scores above):   _____ (A)

No. of questions which actually applied to this article (maximum = 24):   _____ (B)

Maximum possible score (2 × B):   _____ (C)

OVERALL RATING (A/C expressed as a percentage):   _____ %

COMMENTS:

RATING SCALE 5 FOR ARTICLE ON PROGNOSIS

		Yes	Unclear/possibly	No	Not applicable
			Ring the appropriate code		
RESULTS					
1	Is the risk per unit time of the outcome event(s) given?	2	1	0	N/A
2	Is this risk of clinical importance?	2	1	0	N/A
3	Is the estimate of risk sufficiently precise?	2	1	0	N/A
VALIDITY					
Selection					
4	Was the phase of the disease well defined?	2	1	0	N/A
5	Were patients at a uniform point in this phase?	2	1	0	N/A
6	Was the referral pattern described?	2	1	0	N/A
Follow-up					
7	Was follow-up sufficiently complete (under 10% lost to follow-up)?	2	1	0	N/A
8	Were the outcome measurements objective?	2	1	0	N/A
9	Was outcome assessment 'blind'?	2	1	0	N/A
Statistical analysis					
10	Were additional prognostic factors allowed for?	2	1	0	N/A
11	Was validation of the prognostic factor(s) performed?	2	1	0	N/A
12	Were there reasonable numbers of events (10–20 events per prognostic factor)?	2	1	0	N/A
13	Were appropriate methods used?	2	1	0	N/A
14	Were 'unusual' methods justified?	2	1	0	N/A
UTILITY					
15	Do the results help me choose treatments?	2	1	0	N/A
16	Do the results help me reassure/counsel patients?	2	1	0	N/A

TOTAL (add ringed scores above): _____ **(A)**

No. of questions which actually applied to this article (maximum = 16): _____ **(B)**

Maximum possible score (2 × B): _____ **(C)**

OVERALL RATING (A/C expressed as a percentage): _____ %

COMMENTS:

RATING SCALE 6 FOR OVERVIEW ARTICLE

	Ring the appropriate code			
	Yes	Unclear/ possibly	No	Not applicable
RESULTS				
1 Is a summary estimate of association (e.g. odds ratio, relative risk or risk difference) given?	2	1	0	N/A
2 Is this association of clinical importance?	2	1	0	N/A
3 Is the estimate of risk (or relative risk) sufficiently precise?	2	1	0	N/A
VALIDITY				
Selection				
4 Were inclusion criteria for the studies well defined?	2	1	0	N/A
5 Was a well-posed question addressed?	2	1	0	N/A
6 Were convincing efforts made to find all relevant studies?	2	1	0	N/A
7 Was the quality of the studies assessed?	2	1	0	N/A
Statistical analysis				
8 Was the quality of the studies allowed for in the analysis?	2	1	0	N/A
9 Was the quality assessment reproducible?	2	1	0	N/A
10 Was the analysis based on individual patient data?	2	1	0	N/A
11 Were results from each study similar enough to be pooled?	2	1	0	N/A
12 Were sources of variability identified?	2	1	0	N/A
UTILITY				
13 Do the results help me choose a treatment?	2	1	0	N/A
14 Were all clinically important outcomes considered?	2	1	0	N/A

TOTAL (add ringed scores above): _____ **(A)**

No. of questions which actually applied to this article (maximum = 14): _____ **(B)**

Maximum possible score (2 × B): _____ **(C)**

OVERALL RATING (A/C expressed as a percentage): _____ %

COMMENTS:

APPENDIX II Using the literature for evidence based medicine

THE PRACTICE OF EVIDENCE BASED MEDICINE

The practice of evidence based medicine derives from the following premises (Davidoff *et al.*, 1995):

- Clinical decisions should be based on the best available scientific evidence, informed by epidemiological and biostatistical reasoning.

- The clinical problem should determine the type of evidence to be sought.

- Conclusions from identified and critically appraised evidence must lead to changed patient management or health care decisions.

- Clinical performance should be constantly evaluated.

FRAMING THE RESEARCH QUESTION BEHIND THE CLINICAL PROBLEM

In this book, one of our first questions in each of the exercises has been concerned with formulation of the research question arising from the clinical scenario. Readers have been encouraged to **frame the underlying research question** in terms of:

- The kind of patient (age, sex, diagnosis, etc.).

- The intervention, exposure or technique applied to patients.

- The outcome of interest.

The title of a good journal article will usually reflect each of these components

A MEDLINE search of the literature will need to address these three components and it will often be useful to restrict the search to the type of article of interest, for example to randomized controlled trials in the first instance for therapy. The abstract may be searched for words of interest in the text, using an asterisk to ensure that, for example, if we look for 'randomized' we also pick up 'randomize', and 'randomization' by searching for 'random*'. Each citation in MEDLINE has also been classified using a hierarchical classified system of keywords (e.g. RANDOMIZED-CONTROLLED-TRIALS) known as Medical Subject Headings (MESH). This field and over 20 others within the citation, like title, authors, language and publication type, may all be searched, separately or all at once.

The literature search process:

- Identify research question.

- For each component of the research question, identify possible search terms (text words or MESH headings).

- Develop search strategy to further limit the scope of the search.

- Adjust search strategies to broaden the search (if too few articles found) or limit it (if too many).

Search strategy examples:

- Limit to English language.

- Maximize search sensitivity by using highly specific combinations of search terms for the type of article, so that nearly all available articles are found. Typically, using such strategies developed at McMaster University, four or five terms in fields like PT (Publication Type) and Tl (Title) or AB (Abstract) may be used. An example developed at the UK Cochrane Centre uses 34 steps to achieve optimally sensitive searches!

- Maximize search specificity so that irrelevant articles are not found.

KEEPING UP WITH THE LITERATURE

Because medical practitioners cannot hope to keep up with the estimated 6000 articles (Davidoff *et al.*, 1995) on adult general medicine in 20 key medical journals each year (17 articles to read every day), the *ACP Journal Club* condenses 300 articles, selected from the 6000, into a page or so each, instead of four or five. A new journal, *Evidence Based Medicine*, covers some of the same ground as well as general practice, paediatrics, surgery, obstetrics and gynaecology, psychiatry, public health and some anaesthesia. Preference is given to common conditions.

Further reading

Davidoff F, Haynes B, Sackettt D, and Smith R. Evidence Based Medicine: a new journal to help doctors identify the information they need. *Br Med J* 1995; **310:** 1085–1086

Getzsce PC and Lange B. Comparison of search strategies for recalling double-blind trials from Medline. *Dan Med Bull* 1991; **38:** 476–478

Haynes RB *et al.* Developing optimal search strategies for detecting clinically sound studies in MEDLINE. *J Am Med Informat Assoc* 1994; **1:** 447–458

Jadad AR and McQuay HJ. Be systematic in your searching. *Br Med J* 1993; **307:** 66

Jadad AR and McQuay HJ. A high-yield strategy to identify randomised controlled trials for systematic reviews. *Online J Curr Clin Trials* [*serial online*] 1993; Doc No 33: 3973 words; 39 paragraphs

Knipschild P. Systematic reviews: some examples. *Br Med J* 1994; **309:** 719–721

Lefebvre C. Difficulties in identifying articles in MEDLINE using indexing terms (MeSH): experience based on attempts to identify reports of randomized controlled trials. *IFH Healthcare Newsletter* 1994; **3:**(2), 10–15

Lowe HJ and Barnett GO. Understanding and using the Medical Subject Headings (MeSH) vocabulary to perform literature searches. *JAMA* 1994; **271:** 1103–1108

McKibbon KA and Walker CJ. Panning for applied clinical research gold. *Online* 1993; **Jul:** 105–108

McKibbon KA and Walker CJ. Beyond ACP Journal Club: how to harness MEDLINE for diagnosis problems [Editorial]. *ACP J Club* 1994 Sep–Oct: A10 (*Ann Intern Med* 121: Suppl 2)

McKibbon KA and Walker CJ. Beyond ACP Journal Club: how to harness MEDLINE for etiology problems [Editorial]. *ACP J Club* 1994 Nov–Dec: A10–11 (*Ann Intern Med* 121: Suppl 3)

McKibbon KA and Walker CJ. Beyond ACP Journal Club: how to harness MEDLINE for therapy problems [Editorial]. *ACP J Club* 1994 Jul–Aug: A10 (*Ann Intern Med* 121: Suppl 1)

McKibbon KA and Walker-Dilks C. *Evidence-based Health Care for Librarians: panning for gold. How to apply research methodology to search for therapy, diagnosis, etiology, prognosis, review, and meta-analysis articles.* Health Information Research Unit, McMaster University, Ontario, 1995

APPENDIX III Evidence based medicine on the Internet

The Internet provides access to a wealth of resources relating to evidence based medicine (EBM), as well as enabling quick and convenient communication between people with an interest in this area. This section suggests some resources you might like to investigate if you have Internet access.

Only a few places to visit have been suggested, because each site makes available its own comprehensive contents list, as well as suggesting other resources. As is usual with Internet resources, the most up-to-date information on what is available can *only* be found on the Internet!

OUR WORLD WIDE WEB PAGES

We have created some pages on the World Wide Web specifically for readers of this book. The idea of the pages is to give you an easy single reference point to start from if you are exploring the Web for EBM resources, and we hope you will want to pay us a visit.

When you visit the Web pages, you will be able to:

- Give us your comments on this book and your ideas for improvements.

- Enter the scores you gave the papers in the book, and compare your scores with those of other readers.

- Get 'single click' access to a range of important EBM Web sites.

- Find out about other EBM Internet resources which there is not the space to list here.

The address of the Sheffield EBM pages is:

http://www.shef.ac.uk/uni/academic/R-Z/scharr/ebm

OTHER EBM RESOURCES

The Health Information Research Unit at McMaster University in Canada (the 'birthplace' of evidence based medicine) is an important source of materials on EBM. The easiest way to visit is via the Web, at the following address:

http://hiru.mcmaster.ca/ebm/default.htm

The Cochrane Collaboration is an international network of 'health care providers, consumers and scientists' dedicated to the systematic review of all randomized controlled trials of health care. The Cochrane Collaboration handbook, which provides information on conducting systematic reviews of the literature, is available by ftp from:

ftp.cochrane.co.uk (login as anonymous,
with your own email address as the password)

Alternatively, section 1 of the handbook can be found on the World Wide Web at:

http://hiru.mcmaster.ca/cochrane/handbook/cchb_01_.htm

Further general information about the Cochrane Collaboration is available from their pages at:

http.//hiru.mcmaster.ca/cochrane/

In addition, the Centre for Evidence Based Medicine in Oxford maintains a bank of regularly updated educational packages from EBM workshops held in the UK, Norway, Holland, Canada and elsewhere. It is also developing other materials, including a set of interactive programmes for generating, storing and sharing summaries of critically appraised topics ('CATs'). You can access the Centre at:

http://cebm.jr2.ox.ac.uk/

EMAIL DISCUSSION LISTS

An evidence based health care discussion list is run in the UK, via Mailbase, to stimulate discussion, debate and share information about meetings, courses and so on.

When you join a discussion list, you receive the email messages which other members of the list contribute to it, and you can send your own messages to the list, which everyone else then receives. You can join a list without having full Internet access, if you have email access to the net.

To join the evidence based health list, send an email to:

mailbase@mailbase.ac.uk

The only text of your message should be:

join evidence-based-health ⟨ *your first name* ⟩ ⟨ *your last name* ⟩

Index of boxes